S+ Functional Data Analysis

Douglas B. Clarkson
Chris Fraley
Charles C. Gu
James O. Ramsey

S+ Functional Data Analysis

Data Analysis

User's Manual for Windows®

With 79 Illustrations

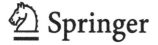 Springer

Douglas B. Clarkson
Insightful Corporation
1700 Westlake Ave. N.
Seattle, WA 98109

Charles C. Gu
Insightful Corporation
1700 Westlake Ave. N.
Seattle, WA 98109

Chris Fraley
Insightful Corporation
1700 Westlake Ave. N.
Seattle, WA 98109

James O. Ramsey
McGill University
1025 Dr. Penfield Ave
Montreal, Quebec H3A 1B1

With 79 illustrations.

Insightful, Insightful Corporation, "Insightful intelligence from data", S-PLUS, S+, S-PLUS Graphlets, Graphlets, and InFact are registered trademarks of Insightful Corporation. Insightful Miner, ArrayAnalyzer, FinMetrics, NuOpt, SeqTrial, Wavelets, and SpatialStats are trademarks of Insightful Corporation. All product names mentioned herein may be trademarks or registered trademarks of their respective companies.

Additional material to this book can be downloaded from http://extras.springer.com

Library of Congress Control Number: 2005924801

ISBN-10 0-387-24969-9   Printed on acid-free paper.
ISBN-13 978-0387-24969-9

(MVA)

9 8 7 6 5 4 3 2 1   11371380

springeronline.com

ACKNOWLEDGMENTS

The software for the Functional Data Analysis module was originally written by Jim Ramsay, Department of Psychology, McGill University, and Bernard Silverman, Department of Mathematics, University of Bristol. We have contributed enhancements and extensions, and attempted to reflect their zeal for the analysis of functional data. We have benefited from contributions by James Schimert, and comments by Tim Hesterberg at Insightful Corporation. Our efforts were funded by NIH SBIR grants 1R43CA86539-01 and 2R44CA86539-02 entitled: *An S-Plus Functional Data Analysis Module.*

CONTENTS

PREFACE

The book is intended as a guide to the functional data analysis software in the S+FDA library. It gives a general overview, and treats each topic through illustrative examples. The code for the examples can be found in the script files provided with the software, which also include additional examples. Users can learn to use the S+FDA library by executing the example scripts while reading. Details on the functions and their arguments, as well as further examples, can be found in the associated help files.

INTRODUCTION

1

Functional data arise in many fields of research. Measurements are often best thought of as functions, even in cases where the data is gathered at a relatively small number of points. Examples include weather changes, stock prices, bone shapes, growth rates, health status indicators, and tumor size.

For time-dependent data, observations may be viewed as realizations of a smooth function $y(t)$ of time that have been measured (with error) at specific time points t_j, but which could have been measured at any time. Spatial functional data is also common, e.g., the length of a bone along an axis, the concentration of a drug in a tissue as a function of depth, yearly mean temperature as a function of location.

Historically, functional data have been analyzed using multivariate or time-series methods at discrete measurement points. Analyzing functional data instead as functions has several advantages:

- Functions, unlike raw data, can be evaluated at any "time" point. This is important because it allows the use of statistical methods requiring evenly-spaced measurements and allows extrapolation for use in predictions or treatment decisions.

- Functional methods (e.g., functional principal components, functional canonical correlation) apply even when the data have been gathered at irregular intervals, or at different times on different subjects, when multivariate analogues of these methods are either inappropriate or unavailable.

- Derivatives and integrals of functions may provide important information about the underlying process. For example, knowledge of the direction and rate of change of a patient's temperature may be more important than knowledge of the patient's current temperature.

Functional methods can also be used when the parameters to be estimated are functions. Ramsay and Silverman (1997) use smoothing spline methods for density estimation, and to estimate the link function in generalized linear models. Another example is regression splines for fitting time-dependent hazard regression models (Kooperberg and Clarkson, 1997).

S+FDA integrates functional data analysis methods into S-PLUS. It includes a complete commercial implementation of the exploratory methods of Ramsay and Silverman (1997, 2002), featuring:

- methods for transforming observed data to a smoothed functional form,

- predicting a functional or nonfunctional variable $y(t)$ as a function of one or more functional or nonfunctional variables,

- finding and rotating the functional "principal components" of a functional variable,

- finding the canonical correlations between two functional variables, and

- performing a "principal differential analysis".

S+FDA also incorporates more recent innovations and extensions, such as allowing the use of functions with arbitrary bases, and providing methods for functional generalized linear models and functional cluster analysis.

Installation

To install the software:

- Go to the website: `http://www.insightful.com/downloads/libraries/default.asp`

- Follow the on-screen Setup instructions; default settings are recommended.

Object-oriented Programming

S+FDA makes use of the object-oriented capabilities of the S-PLUS language. In object-oriented programming, constructor functions create structured data "objects" that are assigned a class (which typically has the same name as the constructor). The object-oriented paradigm allows users to apply generic functions (such as `plot`) to these classed objects, the details of which are handled transparently through class-specific functions or "methods". This simplifies programming by avoiding the need to explicitly invoke different functions or to have additional function arguments when generic operations are applied to objects of different structures.

INTRODUCTORY TUTORIAL (HEIGHT DATA)

We illustrate some exploratory functional data analysis methods using the Berkeley height data (Tuddenham and Snyder, 1954). The corresponding data frame, heightData, is included in the S+FDA library. This data contains the heights of 54 female (columns 2 to 55) and 39 male (columns 56 to 94) children observed at 31 times from age 1 to age 18. The times of measurement are included as the variable age (column 1). We first inspect the data graphically by plotting the height curves as follows:

```
#Set up the plot and label
> plot(heightData$age, heightData[,2], type="n",
        ylim=range(unlist(heightData[,2:55])),
        xlab="Age (years)", ylab="Height (cm)",
        main="Female Height Data")
#draw the height curves
> matlines(heightData$age,as.matrix(heightData[,2:55]))
```

The result is shown in Figure 1.1.

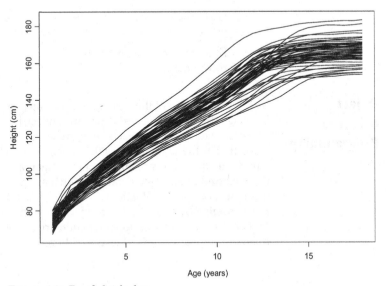

Figure 1.1: *Female height data.*

Although the data appear as smooth curves, only 31 discrete values of height were measured. The curves are produced by connecting these discrete points with straight lines.

As a functional data analysis application, we fit a function to each height curve using linear least squares. The function is represented as a linear combination of basis functions $b_j(t)$ and coefficients β_j that vary from one height function to the next:

$$f(x) = \sum_{j=1}^{n_b} \beta_j b_j(t)$$

There are a variety of choices for the basis functions, e.g., B-splines, Fourier series, and exponential series. Once the basis is chosen, the coefficients are estimated based on the observed data. In Figure 1.1, a *polygonal basis* of connected line segments is used to draw the curves.

Although the functional representation almost always differs from the data at the points of observation, these differences are assumed to be small in the sense that the coefficients β_j capture the information contained in the discretized curve. In most analyses, the raw data is ignored once the β_j have been estimated because it is simpler to work with the functional form. The assumption is that the within-subject variance in the β_j estimates is small compared to the between-subject variance.

Warning

When the number of observations for estimating the β_j is small to moderate or when the within-subject variance of the β_j estimates is large, a mixed-effects model may be preferred so that information may be combined across subjects.

Selecting the Basis Functions

To perform a functional data analysis, we must first choose an appropriate set of basis functions. In the example above, 16 B-spline basis functions of order 6 were used. Since the order of a polynomial basis is the degree plus one, this basis consists of 16 piecewise polynomial splines of degree 5. By default, the *interior* knots for the 16 basis functions are equally spaced over the range of the independent variable (the two *exterior* knots are placed at the endpoints of the function domain). Since height is being viewed as a function of age, the appropriate domain for the basis functions is the age span of the data. The following forms an object of class "bsplineBasis" for the height data:

```
> heightBasis <- bsplineBasis(fDomain
             =range(heightData$age), nbasis=16,norder=6)
```

The basis functions, displayed in Figure 1.2, are equally spaced over the domain:

```
> plot(heightBasis, main="B-spline Basis Functions")
```

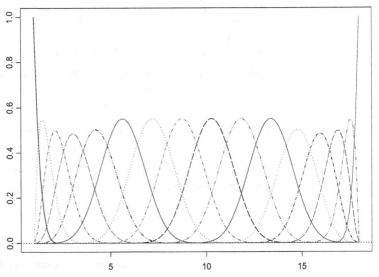

Figure 1.2: *A set of 16 B-spline basis functions.*

Now that we have defined a basis, we need to calculate the coefficients for each height curve. Since there are 93 subjects in this dataset, there should be 93 sets of coefficients (one set for each function). The S+FDA function fVector takes the basis, the data matrix, and the independent variable, and returns an object of class "fVector" containing the linear least-squares estimates of the coefficients. An "fVector" object has two additional attributes:

"basis", which stores the basis used in the fit, and "fNames", which stores labeling information for the data. In the code below, we also specify names for the independent variable (age), the subjects (child), and the units of the response (height). These names are used in the plotting and printing functions.

```
> fHgt <- fVector(object=heightBasis, y=heightData[,2:94],
            fArgs=heightData$age,
            fNames=list(age=heightData$age,
            child=names(heightData)[2:94], height='cm'))
```

Extract the estimated coefficients, basis functions, and function names from fHgt using the commands getCoef(fHgt), getBasis(fHgt), and getNames(fHgt), respectively.

Smoothing

Although the basis functions smooth the curves, additional smoothing may be beneficial. The S-PLUS functions for creating functional data objects allow specification of a smoothing penalty in the least-squares objective. The penalty also requires a smoothing parameter, lambda. You may estimate an optimal lambda by minimizing a generalized cross validation statistic. See section Generalized Cross Validation on page 82 for more details.

Smoothing techniques are largely exploratory in nature, and are discussed in more detail in Chapter 4 of this manual, as well as in Chapter 4 of Ramsay and Silverman (1997). We will have occasion to use smoothing techniques for most of the functional data analysis methods provided in S+FDA.

As an example, penalize the squared second derivative with a penalty parameter lambda=0.001:

```
> fHgt2 <- fVector(object=heightBasis,
            y=heightData[, 2:94], fArgs=heightData$age,
            penalty=list(lambda=0.001, linDop=fDop(2)),
            fNames=list(age=heightData$age,
            child=names(heightData)[2:94], height='cm'))
```

Compare with the original data of Figure 1.1 to see how closely the smoothed functions fit the data. The S-PLUS function fEval evaluates an object of class "fVector" at any point in the domain of the basis. Here, we evaluate the 54 spline curves for the females at the original age values (heightData$age), calculate the difference between predicted and observed heights, and then plot the curve differences at the given ages:

```
> hgtFemale<-fEval(fHgt2[1:54], heightData$age)

> plot(heightData$age, hgtFemale[,1], type="n",
        ylim=range(hgtFemale-as.matrix(heightData[,2:55])),
        xlab="Age (years)", ylab="Height Difference (cm)",
        main="Female Height Differences with Splines")
> matpoints(heightData$age,
        hgtFemale-as.matrix(heightData[, 2:55]), pch="o")
```

The resulting plot is given in Figure 1.3.

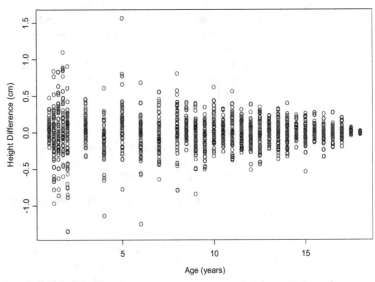

Figure 1.3: *Difference between predicted and actual female height data when using cubic B-splines for function representation.*

The maximum deviation between the spline approximation and the true heights is about 1.5 cm compared with height values of 80 cm or more (see Figure 1.1). These differences are small enough that we consider the smoothed functions to be acceptable for subsequent analysis.

Given a representation of the data as an fVector object, it is easy to conduct several kinds of exploratory analyses with S+FDA. Here, we compute the first two derivatives of height with respect to time. We begin with the first derivative:

```
> plot(fVector(fHgt2[1:54], linDop = fDop(1)),
        xlab="age (years)",
        ylab="First Derivative of Height (cm/year)",
        main="Female Height, First Derivative")
```

The result is displayed in Figure 1.4.

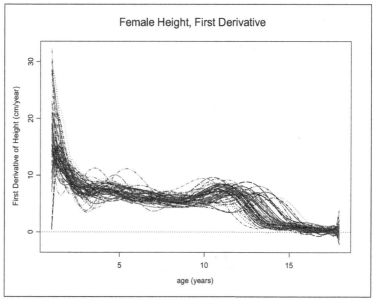

Figure 1.4: *First derivatives of the functional representation of the female height data. The second derivative was penalized for smoothing, with penalty parameter 0.001.*

Despite the large number of curves in Figure 1.4, some general trends are apparent: there appears to be an acceleration in growth around age 4, with a second acceleration after age 10. Further exploratory analysis, such as plotting the mean of the 54 derivative functions, may help reveal more structure.

The plot of the second derivatives is produced in a similar fashion:

9

```
> plot(fVector(fHgt2[1:54], linDop=fDop(2)),
    xlab="Age (years)",
    ylab="Second Derivative of Height (cm/year^2)",
    main="Female Height, Second Derivative")
```

The result is displayed in Figure 1.5.

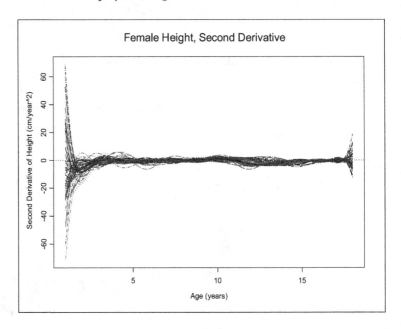

Figure 1.5: *Second derivatives of the functional representation of the female height data. The second derivative was penalized for smoothing, with penalty parameter 0.001.*

The large function values near the endpoints in both derivative plots are due to lack of information concerning values outside the interval. Smoothing by penalizing a higher derivative would reduce the variation at the endpoints, although possibly at the risk of oversmoothing the function. Such considerations are discussed in more detail in the chapter on smoothing.

Because we use splines of degree five (order 6) when fitting the functions, the second derivatives are smooth, cubic splines. Had we fit the raw data with cubic splines (order 4), the second derivative curves would have been piecewise linear. In general, if an analysis requires a smooth kth derivative, and smoothness in higher derivatives is unimportant, splines of degree k+3 (order k+4) should be used to fit the functions so that the kth derivative will be a cubic spline.

The ease with which you can examine the derivatives is a direct consequence of the functional approach, and one of its main advantages. By regarding the height measurements for each person as a smooth curve, you are no longer constrained by discrete observation times.

A LINEAR MODEL FOR THE HEIGHT DATA

Now consider a functional linear model for predicting sex in terms of the growth rate, the first derivative of the height curve. Since the dependent variable is binary, this model can also be considered a discriminant function for predicting sex in terms of the growth rate.

For the height data, fit a functional linear model as follows:

```
> predLm <- fLM(sex~-1+fVector(fHgt, linDop=fDop(1)),
                data.frame(fHgt=fHgt,
                sex=c(rep(1,54), rep(0,39))))
```

Here the -1 in the model formula eliminates the intercept, which is already contained in the B-splines. The coefficients in the resulting model are functional. The first coefficient estimate may be plotted as follows:

```
> plot(predLm$coef[[1]], xlab="age", ylab="beta",
       main="Coefficient Function")
```

The resulting plot is shown in Figure 1.6.

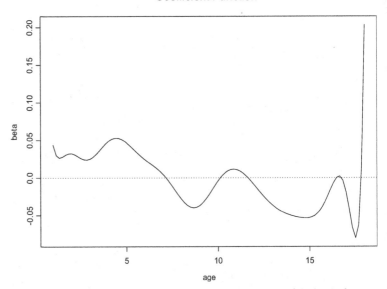

Figure 1.6: *The function of coefficients predicting sex in terms of the height function.*

The effect of the growth rate on the linear model prediction has a maximum around age 5, is positive again at around age 11, and is negative during the puberty growth spurt after age 11. The negative lobe after age 11 predicts maleness, when the boys have their growth spurts, but the girls are finished theirs.

To see how well the resulting model can discriminate between males and females, plot the fitted values:

```
> score <- getCoef(predLm$fitted.values)
> plot(as.factor(c(rep("F",54),rep("M",39))),
      score, main="Linear Model Predicted Values")
```

The results are displayed in Figure 1.7.

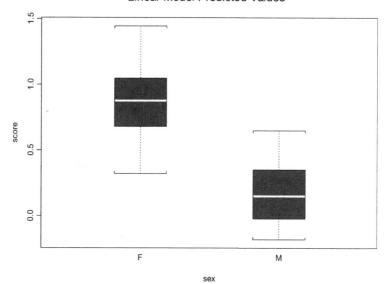

Figure 1.7: *Predicted height scores for each sex*

Most females have a score above 0.5, and most males have a score below 0.5, so that growth rates are an effective means of classifying the observations.

Discussion   In this simple example of a functional linear model, we have again used derivative information, this time to predict the sex of the individual. Although the results for this example are good, generally predictions based on functional linear models should be viewed with caution. When the independent variable is functional, so are the coefficient estimates, and outliers may significantly influence the outcome (overfitting). Methods to avoid overfitting, particularly smoothing methods, are discussed in more detail in the chapter on functional linear models.

CLUSTER ANALYSIS OF THE HEIGHT DATA

One approach to cluster analysis is to search for natural groups of observations by examining "distances" between observations. For the height data discussed in the previous section, clustering can be based on a Euclidean or other distance measure between the observed heights at the observation times (the ages). Specifying these distances requires that all individuals be measured at the same times. This requirement can be met by first converting the observed data to functional form. Once this is accomplished, a much broader class of distance measures becomes available. For example, derivatives can be incorporated into the distance metrics. For the height data, we might be interested in patterns of growth curves related to the growth rate (the velocity, i.e., first derivative) or the rate of change in the growth rate (the acceleration, i.e., second derivative). If, for example, our main interest is the growth rate, then we could define the distance between the growth curve functions $f_1(t)$ and $f_2(t)$ for two individuals as the square root of the integrated squared distance between the first derivatives of the two height curves:

$$d(f_1(t), f_2(t)) = \sqrt{\int_t \left(\frac{df_1(t)}{dt} - \frac{df_2(t)}{dt} \right)^2 dt}$$

This distance measurement is based on the rate of change of growth, as opposed to the final height achieved.

Computing a Distance Matrix

For the clustering example, we consider only the height data starting from age 3. The reason for this is that the data in infancy are unstable, and the transition to standing height around age 2 introduces a significant perturbation. We recompute the smoothed fHgt from age 3:

```
> ageRange <- heightData$age >= 3
> heightBasis <- bsplineBasis(fDomain
                     =range(heightData$age[ageRange]),
                     nbasis=16, norder=6)
> fHgt3 <- fVector(object=heightBasis,
```

```
y=heightData[ageRange,2:94],
fArgs=heightData$age[ageRange],
penalty=list(lambda=0.001, linDop=fDop(2)),
fNames=list(age=heightData$age[ageRange],
            child=names(heightData)[2:94],
            height='cm'))
```

The choice of lambda=0.001 is determined by a procedure described in section Generalized Cross Validation on page 82 .

The S+FDA function fDist computes distance matrices from functional data. The following S-PLUS code computes a distance matrix whose (i, j) element contains the square root of the integrated squared distance between the first derivatives of growth functions (i) and (j) for the height data:

```
> distHgt <- sqrt(fDist(fHgt3, linDop=fDop(1)))
```

Now we can apply any clustering method based on distance matrices. For example, the S-PLUS function hclust computes clusters for a variety of hierarchical clustering methods from a distance matrix. Here we use average-linkage clustering:

```
> clustHgt <- hclust(distHgt, method="average")
```

A plot of the cluster tree label according to sex is obtained as follows:

```
> sex <- as.factor(c(rep("F", 54), rep("M", 39)))
> plclust(clustHgt, labels=as.character(sex))
```

The result is displayed in Figure 1.8:

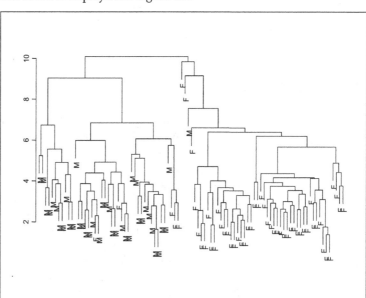

Figure 1.8: *Complete linkage cluster tree labeled according to sex.*

Displaying the Cluster Mean Functions

Since we have heights for both males and females, it would seem natural to group the data by sex. The labeling in Figure 1.8 shows that this grouping is supported by the cluster analysis, indicating that males and females generally have different growth patterns. Only one male appears in the female subtree, and relatively few females appear in the male subtree. To investigate this further, we apply the S-PLUS function cutree to obtain the two-group solution:

```
> g <- 2
> groupsHgt <- cutree(clustHgt, k=g)
```

The clusters are as defined by a horizontal line at about distance 9.5 in Figure 1.8. The frequency of males and females in each of the groups is easily obtained using the S-PLUS function crosstabs:

```
> crosstabs(~groupsHgt+sex)
```

for which an abbreviated output is shown below:

```
         |F       |M       |RowTotl|
- - - - - - - + - - - - - - - + - - - - - - - + - - - - - - - +
  1      |49      | 1       |50      |
- - - - - - - + - - - - - - - + - - - - - - - + - - - - - - - +
  2      | 5      |38       |43      |
- - - - - - - + - - - - - - - + - - - - - - - + - - - - - - - +
 ColTotl|54      |39       |93      |
- - - - - - - + - - - - - - - + - - - - - - - + - - - - - - - +
```

Group 1 is predominantly female and group 2 predominantly male. We split the data into a list grouped by cluster, and plot the function and derivative means for each group:

```
> splitGroups <- split(fHgt3, groupsHgt)
> par(mfrow=c(2,1))
> plot(1, 20, type="n", xlab="age", ylab="height",
        main="Group Mean Function Heights",
        xlim=c(0, 19), ylim=c(60,200))
> temp <- lapply(1:g, function(i)
            lines(mean(splitGroups[[i]]), lty=i, col=i))
> legend(1, 190, paste(1:g), col=1:g, lty=1:g)
> plot(15, 20, type="n", xlab="age", ylab="height",
        main="Group Mean Derivative Heights",
        xlim=c(0, 19), ylim=c(0,30))
> temp <- lapply(1:g, function(i)
                lines(mean(fVector(splitGroups[[i]],
                    linDop=fDop(1)))), lty=i))
> legend(15, 29, paste(1:g), col=1:g,
            lty=1:g, background=0)
```

The results are shown in Figure 1.9. Since derivatives were used to define the distances, one would expect cluster differences to be reflected in their means, shown in the lower half of Figure 1.9. The display shows that the behavior of the clusters differs with respect to the time and duration of the growth spurt around puberty. There is also a difference in the groups around age 5 where group 1 (mostly females) tends to have a minor growth spurt that is not present in mostly-male group 2.

Between Cluster Distances

Hierarchical clustering methods produce a grouping for a given number of clusters, but do not include a mechanism for selecting the correct number of clusters. The choice of two groups was based on informal inspection of the clustering tree (Figure 1.8). Because of the small number of cross-overs from males to females, the two-group solution (males versus females) would seem satisfactory. However, if the labeling according to sex were not available, we would be unlikely to reach this conclusion.

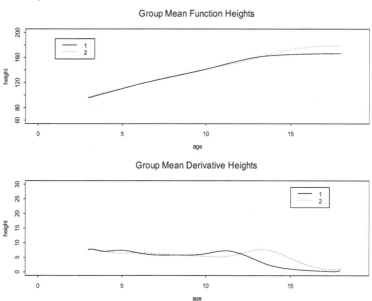

Figure 1.9: *The mean function (top) and its first derivative for the two groups in Figure 1.8*

Summary

This clustering example illustrates the flexibility of functional data analysis methods - when the data are thought of as functions, distance measures based on derivatives are possible, and derivatives can be used to analyze group structure.

Multidimensional Scaling

Multidimensional scaling is also possible once a distance matrix is available. We applied the S-PLUS function cmdscale to the distance matrix (using the command cmdscale(distHgt)) to do a simple multidimensional scaling analysis. In a plot of the (two dimensional) solution (not shown), the males and females are well separated.

The S+FDA library offers many other methods for functional data analysis. These are discussed more fully in subsequent chapters, as well as in Ramsay and Silverman (1997, 2002).

FDA FLOW CHART

The flowchart in Figure 1.10 represents the organization of this manual.

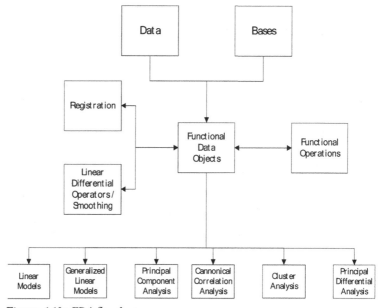

Figure 1.10: *FDA flowchart.*

Each box in the flowchart represents a chapter. Functional data analysis begins by selecting a basis to represent discrete data in functional form. The data typically correspond to a sample of functions, so that *registration* to remove unimportant differences (e.g. phase and/or amplitude variations) between samples may be necessary. Although the basis representation usually provides some smoothing, it is often desirable to apply one or more smoothing operations before analysis. This smoothing may be accomplished via a penalty on a linear differential operator applied to the functions.

Once a functional data object has been created, it can be analyzed and transformed in ways that are not possible for discrete data. You may perform various arithmetic operations, including differentiation and integration. In addition, a variety of analyses from discrete data analysis have functional analogs: linear and generalized linear

21

generalized linear modeling, principal component and canonical correlation analysis, and cluster analysis. Principal differential analysis, which has no analog for discrete data, is another option for functional data.

BASIS OBJECTS AND OPERATIONS

2

WHAT IS A BASIS?

Univariate   In the S+FDA library, univariate functions are represented as linear combinations of basis functions:

$$f(x) = \sum_{j=1}^{n_b} \beta_j b_j(x)$$

where the β_j are coefficients, and the b_j are known basis functions. For example, in an exponential basis, $b_j(t) = \exp(k_j t)$ for user-specified parameters k_j.

Bivariate   Similarly, bivariate functions may be represented as:

$$f(x, y) = \sum_{j=1}^{n_b} \beta_j b_j(x, y)$$

where $b_j(x, y)$ are the basis functions based on (triangle) finite elements.

Alternatively, by assuming that the basis functions are *separable*, the representation is:

$$f(x, y) = \sum_{i=1}^{n_x} \sum_{j=1}^{n_y} \beta_{ij} b^x_i(x) b^y_j(y)$$

BASIS OBJECTS

S+FDA supports both univariate and bivariate basis functions including:

- univariate bases: B-spline, Fourier series, polynomial, polygonal, exponential. Moreover, users can define their own bases, and composite bases of two or more bases are also possible.

- bivariate bases: finite element, or the product of two univariate bases.

Univariate

In S+FDA, each of the supported univariate bases is a class that inherits from a larger class called fBasis. Different subclasses of fBasis are defined by the number of basis functions and the domain. Once the user specifies the type of basis, the number of basis functions, and the domain, a basis-specific constructor function computes values for the coefficients from the data.

Bivariate

In S+FDA, the basis may be assumed to be separable, in which case it is the product of two univariate bases functions, and is of class fProdBasis.

If the finite element basis is used, the class is fFinElemBasis.

CHOOSING A UNIVARIATE BASIS

Selecting basis functions is perhaps the most important step in a functional data analysis: the basis functions need to have features as close as possible to the data they estimate so that an accurate representation of the function can be obtained with only a few basis terms.

fSelectBasis

Basis selection is so important that we provide the user with a function called fSelectBasis that is specifically designed for this task. Input to fSelectBasis includes information on whether the function is periodic, how many events are likely to occur in the basis, and whether or not derivatives are needed. Although fSelectBasis function can help in selecting a basis, there is no fully automatic way to select a good basis and knowledge of the problem and available data is of critical importance. Note also that fSelectBasis allows access to only some of the types of bases that are available in the S+FDA library.

Function Properties

The number of events or features that occur in a function is a measure of its complexity. Features or events can be viewed graphically and include peaks, valleys, zero crossings, plateaus, and linear slopes. In the S+FDA function fSelectBasis, if there is only one event, it is assumed that the basis is constant over all values of its domain, with value equal to the value of the single event (class constantBasis). On the other hand, if more than one event is specified and derivatives are required, then a polynomial basis (class bsplineBasis) is used with the number of basis functions equal to the number of events. Finally, if derivatives are not needed, then a piecewise linear spline (class polygonalBasis) can be used.

A function is *periodic* if its values are repeated in fixed intervals. For example, a function that varies in a regular pattern from day to day (e.g., temperature) or over the course of a year (e.g., mean daily temperature) can be thought of as periodic. A periodic function can often be expressed as a *Fourier* series, which is a sum of sine and cosine functions.

Once a set of basis functions has been selected, coefficients must still be estimated. Values of the coefficients vary not only with the underlying data, but also with the fitting procedure. In particular, smoothing techniques may be needed to mitigate the influence of outliers and avoid overfitting. Smoothing is discussed in more detail in Chapter 4.

CHOOSING A BIVARIATE BASIS

In bivariate analysis, the user must decide whether to assume that the basis functions are separable. If so, the product basis function is appropriate. Otherwise, the finite element basis is preferred. The relative advantages of each type are:

- Product: saves computation.

- Finite Element: theoretically more accurate, feasible to differentiate.

See Chapter for a comparison of computation times and accuracy of approximation...

CREATING UNIVARIATE BASES

In object-oriented programming, a constructor for an object usually has the same name as the class assigned to the object. This convention is followed for objects of class fBasis. For example, the function FourierBasis constructs an object of class FourierBasis, and the function bsplineBasis constructs an object of class bsplineBasis. The following section gives more detail on the basis functions available in S+FDA. The description is largely non-mathematical, but is hopefully sufficient to enable you to choose your own basis.

constantBasis The simplest bases are those of class constantBasis. The basis functions in this class are constant (and equal to one) over their entire domain. There is only one argument to the constructor, the domain of the function. The basis may be constructed and plotted using the following commands:

```
> basis <- constantBasis(fDomain=c(0,10))
> plot(basis)
```

The resulting plot is shown in Figure 2.1.

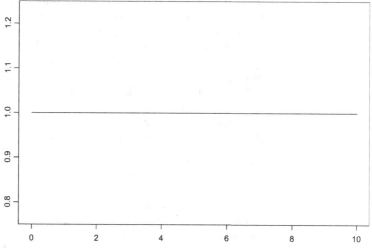

Figure 2.1: *Constant basis function over the domain (0,10).*

The constantBasis constructor is surprisingly useful. Measurements on subjects that do not change with time (e.g., sex) can be included in functional models as functions with a constant basis. Indeed, linear regression models can be viewed as functional linear models in which the basis functions are constant.

bsplineBasis

Piecewise polynomial splines consist of smoothly joined polynomials, where each polynomial is defined between two values called *knots*. In piecewise polynomials, function values of polynomials defined in adjacent intervals are constrained to be equal at the knots, and smoothness is obtained by constraining derivatives to be equal at the knots as well. In B-splines of order k (see, e.g., deBoor, 1978, or Green and Silverman, 1994), derivatives of order up to $k - 1$ are required to be equal at the knots in adjacent polynomials. The *order* of a B-spline is one more than the degree of the piecewise polynomials used in the fit. Thus, an order 4 B-spline is a piecewise cubic (degree 3) polynomial in which the values of the first and second derivatives, in addition to the function values, match at the knots. B-splines are usually preferred over piecewise polynomials because they give a smoother fit to the data.

The bsplineBasis constructor allows as input the domain of the function, the order of the spline, the number of B-spline basis functions, and the location of the knots (although not all of these are needed since, for example, the number of knots and the order of the spline determine the number of basis functions). Ramsay and Silverman (1997) recommend that the order of the spline to be at least as high as the highest-order derivative of interest plus three (or, equivalently, that the degree of the spline be equal to the number of desired derivatives plus two). Using this rule, the highest-order derivative of interest would be a smooth cubic spline.

Knots should be placed appropriately around features in the function such as maxima and minima, with fewer knots in locations where the function shows little variability. The exact knot location is not usually important, but using too few knots may lead to significant error in the functional representation, while using too many knots may lead to overfitting of the data. One common practice is to use a fixed grid of (many) knots, and then apply smoothing methods (see Chapter 4) to eliminate problems due to overfitting. An alternative is to use regression methods to find "optimal" knot locations (see, e.g., Friedman and Silverman, 1989). Currently only the smoothing methods are supported in S+FDA.

The follow constructs and plots the functions in a B-spline basis:

```
> basis <- bsplineBasis(fDomain=c(0,10), norder=6,
                        nbasis=20)
> plot(basis)
```

The resulting plot is given in Figure 2.2.

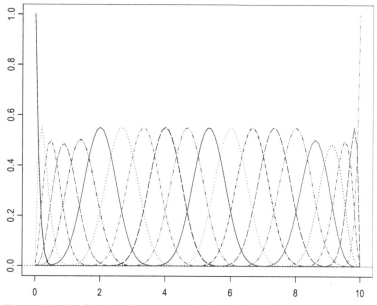

Figure 2.2: *B-spline basis functions over the domain (0,10).*

FourierBasis Periodic functions such as time series are represented by objects of class FourierBasis. Functions represented in this basis have expansions of the following form:

$$f(t) = \beta_0 + \beta_1 \sin \omega t + \beta_2 \cos \omega t + \beta_3 \sin 2\omega t + \beta_4 \cos 2\omega t + \ldots$$

The basis functions are $b_o(t) = 1$, $b_1(t) = \sin \omega t$, $b_2(t) = \cos \omega t$, $b_3(t) = \sin 2\omega t$, etc. The first basis function is a constant, the second a sine function, the third a cosine function with the same period, and so on.

In a Fourier basis there are always an odd number of basis functions, and the period is taken to be the same as the domain of the function. The basis functions are estimated using a fast Fourier transform. A plot of an object of class FourierBasis can be obtained as follows:

```
> basis <- FourierBasis(fDomain=c(0,10), nbasis=4)
> plot(basis)
```

The result is shown in Figure 2.3.

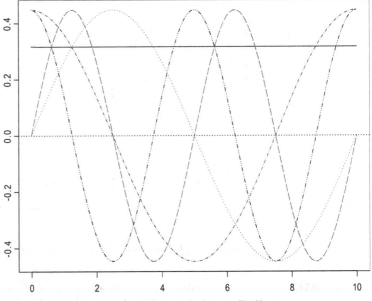

Figure 2.3: *Fourier basis functions over the domain (0,10).*

Notice that although four basis functions were specified, we obtained five basis functions. This is because a Fourier basis always has an odd number of basis functions: the constant basis function plus an equal number of sin and cos basis functions.

polynomialBasis The basis functions in an object of class `polynomialBasis` are the terms of a polynomial centered at a fixed scalar c, for example:

$$p(t) = \beta_0 + \beta_1(t-c) + \beta_2(t-c)^2 + \beta_3(t-c)^3 + \beta_4(t-c)^4$$

The number of basis functions is equal to the degree of the polynomial, plus one. In the polynomial shown, the number of basis functions is five, one for each term in the polynomial.

A plot of the first five functions in a polynomial basis over the domain $(0,10)$ and centered at 5 is obtained as follows (see Figure 2.4):

```
> basis <- polynomialBasis(fDomain=c(0,10),nbasis=5,ctr=5)
> plot(basis)
```

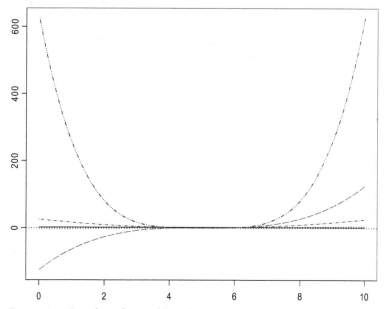

Figure 2.4: *First five polynomial basis functions centered at 5 over domain (0,10).*

Note that any smooth function can be represented by a polynomial basis expansion, since the terms are those of its power series about a point. Unfortunately, the basis functions in polynomial bases tend to be highly correlated and often exhibit numerical instability. Also, the fit may be poor away from the center c, and adaptation to local features removed from c may not be possible without a very large number of basis functions. Although polynomial bases play an important role in classical analysis, they have been superseded by the more flexible B-spline bases in applications.

polygonalBasis   Objects of class `polygonalBasis` are piecewise linear, equivalent to an order 2 (linear) B-spline basis. This basis has the advantage of simplicity, and the disadvantage that the first derivatives are step functions. The `polygonalBasis` constructor has a single argument, `fArgs`, containing the points at which the function changes (the knots in a linear B-spline basis). Perhaps the most common way to use a polygonal basis is to set the knots in `fArgs` equal to the observation times of the function so that the unsmoothed function linearly interpolates the observed data. Smoothing is then used to prevent overfitting.

A plot of five polygonal basis functions is obtained as follows (see Figure 2.5):

```
> basis <- polygonalBasis(fArgs=seq(0, 10, length=5))
> plot(basis)
```

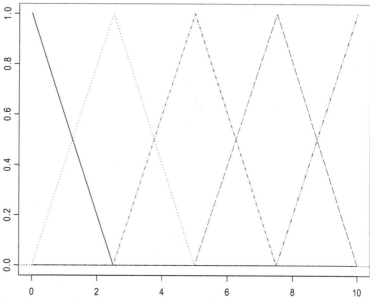

Figure 2.5: *Polygonal basis functions on the domain (0, 10).*

exponentialBasis Objects of class exponentialBasis consist of terms of the form $\exp(k_i t)$ where the k_i are user-specified rate constants. As with polynomial bases away from their center, exponential bases do not adapt well away from the origin. For this reason, exponential bases should only be chosen in special circumstances. A plot of five exponential basis functions is obtained as follows (see Figure 2.6):

```
> basis <- exponentialBasis(fDomain=c(0, 10),
                    ratevec=c(-2, -1, -0.5, -0.25, -0.1))
```

```
> plot(basis)
```

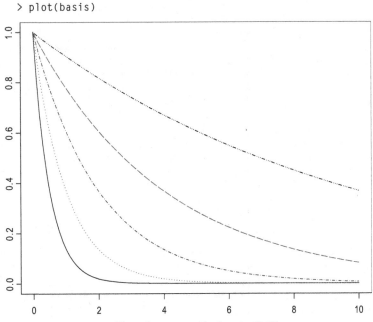

Figure 2.6: *Exponential basis functions on the domain (0,10).*

compositeBasis Objects of class `compositeBasis` represent bases whose terms are selected from one or more fundamental bases. A composite basis is a sum of terms of the form:

$$b_k(x) \;=\; \sum_{j=1}^{n_b} \beta_{kj} b_{kj}(x)$$

each of which is a basis expansion. The following is an example of the representation of a function in terms of a composite basis consisting of three different fundamental bases:

$$f(x) \;=\; \sum_{j=1}^{n_1} \beta_{1j} b_{1j}(x) + \sum_{j=1}^{n_2} \beta_{2j} b_{2j}(x) + \sum_{j=1}^{n_3} \beta_{3j} b_{3j}(x)$$

(there are n_k basis functions of the kth type in this composite basis).

The advantage of a composite basis is the ability to adapt to more complex functions with fewer basis functions. As a simple example, consider a time series with a baseline and a linear trend in time. Such a function can be represented by the composite of a polynomial basis with two terms (a constant plus a linear term) to account for the linear trend, and a Fourier basis to represent the detrended time series.

In a more complex example of a composite basis, we use a constant basis to account for a baseline, an exponential basis to account for exponential decay, and a Fourier basis to account for periodic behavior. Such a basis can be constructed as follows:

```
> basis1 <- constantBasis(fDomain=c(0, 10))
> basis2 <- exponentialBasis(fDomain=c(0, 10), ratevec=-1)
> basis3 <- FourierBasis(fDomain=c(0, 10))
> basis <- compositeBasis(basis1, basis2, basis3)
> plot(basis)
```

The resulting plot is shown in Figure 2.7.

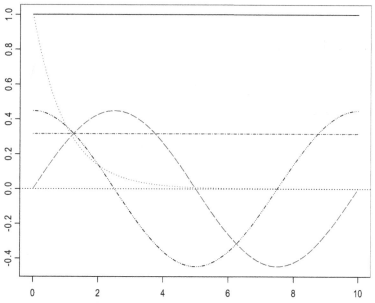

Figure 2.7: *A composite basis consisting of a constant, an exponential decay, and a Fourier series over the domain (0, 10).*

Although we explicitly included a constant basis for a baseline (mean) term, in fact a constant basis functions is already included in the Fourier basis.

CREATING BIVARIATE BASES

Separable Bases

An S-PLUS constructor function `fProdBasis` creates product basis functions for bivariate functional data. Simply supply the two univariate bases that form the product.

For example, to create a product basis consisting of a Fourier and a B-spline univariate basis:

```
> basis1 <- FourierBasis(fDomain=c(0,365), nbasis=11)
> basis2 <- bsplineBasis(fDomain=c(0,52), nbasis=20)
> basisProd <- fProdBasis(basis1, basis2)
```

The result is an object of class `fProdBasis`, which contains as two components the univariate bases:

```
> names(basisProd)
[1] "basis1" "basis2"
```

Finite Element Bases

An S-PLUS constructor function `fFinElemBasis` creates finite element basis functions for bivariate functional data.

```
> args(fFinElemBasis)

function(xDomain, yDomain, params)
```

For example:

```
> basisFinElem <- fFinElemBasis(c(0, 10), c(0, 10),
                                    c(10, 10))
> basisFinElem

Linear Basis for 2D Finite Element Method:

Domain x: 0 10
       y: 0 10

Number of Basis: 121
Number of Element: 200
```

The result is an object of class `fFinElemBasis` which contains the following components:

```
> names(basisFinElem)
```

```
[1] "fDomain"    "Vnode"    "Velem"    "basis.coe"
```

The plot method for the object of class fFinElemBasis is also available for graphic view of the i-th basis function, as shown in Figure 2.8:

```
> plot(basisFinElem)
```

By default, the method picks one basis function in the middle of the domain. In this example, it chooses the 60th basis function.

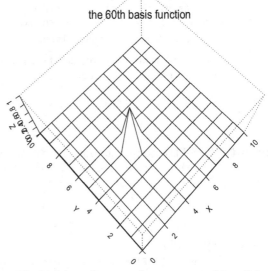

Figure 2.8: *The 60th basis function of* basis2D, *an object of class* fFinElement.

OPERATIONS ON UNIVARIATE BASES

Derivatives

The function fEval produces values of basis functions and their derivatives (when applicable).

Applied to an object that inherits from class fBasis, the required input to fEval includes the basis object, the points at which the basis is to be evaluated, and the desired order of the derivative. The output is the evaluated derivative (or function value) for all basis functions at the specified points.

As an example, evaluate and plot the first derivatives of the exponential basis (displayed in Figure 2.6) over a sequence of numbers of length 100 over the domain (0, 10) using code:

```
> basis <- exponentialBasis(fDomain=c(0,10),
                            ratevec=c(-2, -1, -0.5, -0.25, -0.1))
> dBasis <- fEval(basis, fArg=seq(0, 10, length=100),
                  linDop=fDop(1))
> matplot(seq(0, 10, length=100), dBasis, type="l")
```

The resulting plot is given in Figure 2.9.

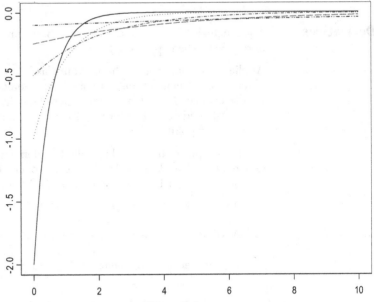

Figure 2.9: *First derivatives of Figure 2.6.*

Integrals

It is also possible to integrate the basis functions. The function fInt integrates all of the functions in a basis over a specified range. For example, the exponential basis in Figure 2.6 can be integrated as follows:

```
> basis <- exponentialBasis(fDomain=c(0,10),
                  ratevec=c(-2, -1, -0.5, -0.25, -0.1))
> fInt(basis, limits=c(0, 10))
```

This results in the following vector of integral values:

```
1.000 0.999 0.999 0.999 0.998 0.994 0.981 0.950 0.864 0.632
```

It is often less computationally expensive to integrate the basis functions over a specified range, and then use these integrals to evaluate the integrals of the functions of interest.

Inner Products   Inner products of basis functions are required in many of the analyses provided in S+FDA. These inner products are integrals of the form:

$$\int b_1(s)b_2(s)ds$$

for any two basis functions $b_1(s)$ and $b_2(s)$, where the two bases are assumed to have the same domain and the integration is over the entire domain. For example, inner products of the basis functions within a particular basis are computed using the function fInProd as follows:

```
> fInProd(basis, basis)
```

The result is a square matrix containing the inner products with dimension equal to the number of functions in basis. This inner product matrix is used, for example, in functional regression models. Inner products of the derivatives of basis functions are also possible.

OPERATIONS ON BIVARIATE BASES

Derivatives

Evaluating bivariate basis functions of class `fFinElemBasis` and their derivatives (when applicable) are the main operations of interest. Integrals of functions are not calculated as the linear combination of the integrals of basis functions, therefore S+FDA does not implement integrals of basis functions.

Evaluate the basis functions at specified arguments by

```
> fEval(basis, fArg1, fArg2=fArg1, xDeriv=0, yDeriv=0)
```

where arguments `xDeriv` and `yDeriv` can be specified by 1 for the first order derivative on x and y. It returns a matrix of basis function values $\beta_s(x_j, y_j)$ with $s = 1, ..., nBasis$ and $j = 1, ...nPoint$.

FUNCTIONAL DATA OBJECTS AND OPERATIONS

3

S+FDA supports functional data objects of either one or two arguments, as described below.

Univariate Functional Data Objects

Univariate functional data objects are represented by objects of class fFunction in S+FDA. Their structure is defined in terms of a basis expansion:

$$f(x) = \sum_{j=1}^{n} \beta_j b_j(x)$$

for known or estimated coefficients β_j and basis functions $b_j(x)$, as discussed in Chapter 2.

Bivariate Functional Data

Functional data objects with two arguments are represented in S+FDA in one of two ways, depending on whether the basis expansion is *separable*. The class of the object is either:

- fProdFunction (for separable basis expansions), or
- fFinElemFunction (for finite element basis expansions).

Separable basis expansions for bivariate functions have the form

$$f(x, y) = \sum_{i=1}^{n_x} \sum_{j=1}^{n_y} \beta_{ij} b_i^x(x) b_j^y(y)$$

where the β_{ij} are known or estimated coefficients, and $b_i^x(x)$ and $b_j^y(y)$ are basis functions from the x and y bases, respectively. With this form, each bivariate function can be written as an inner product of two univariate basis functions. These occur most often in variances computations for vectors of function objects.

More generally, bivariate functions can be expanded as:

$$f(x, y) = \sum_{j=1}^{n_b} \beta_j \Phi_j(x, y)$$

where the β_{ij} are estimated coefficients, $\Phi_j(x, y)$ are *finite element* basis functions. Currently, this expansion is implemented only for linear combinations of the basis functions, not higher order powers of the basis functions.

UNIVARIATE FUNCTIONAL DATA OBJECTS (PINCH FORCE EXAMPLE)

In this section we first describe the various constructors associated with univariate functional data objects in S+FDA, and then discuss some of the most useful operations associated with these objects. Smoothing operations are discussed in the next Chapter.

Constructing Univariate Functional Data Objects

An object of class fFunction represents a single univariate function. It may be constructed using a class fFunction constructor in one of three ways:

- from data -- i.e., a vector of known function values, the arguments at which the functions are evaluated and a basis, or

- from known basis coefficients and the corresponding basis, or

- from an fFunction object or an fVector object with length of 1.

These methods are now discussed in more detail.

Constructing from data and a basis

You may construct an S+FDA object of class fFunction from an object of class fBasis, together with a vector of known function values (observations) and the vector of points at which the function is evaluated.

As an example, we consider a dataset measuring the pinch force of an individual over time (see Ramsay and Silverman, 1997). Individuals pinch a measuring device for about one third of a second, and the force of the pinch is measured. Twenty pinches, each with 151 measurements over time, were observed.

The S+FDA data set pinchmat contains this data, with the columns indexing the replicates and the rows indexing the observed pinch force at each of the 151 observation times. The vector pinchtime contains the 151 times, scaled as a sequence of integers from 0 to 150.

You may create an object of class fFunction using the first column in pinchmat as follows:

```
#Create a basis
> basis <- bsplineBasis(fDomain=range(pinchtime))
#Create an fFunction object
```

```
> onePinch <- fFunction(object=basis, y=pinchmat[,1],
                        fArgs=pinchtime, fNames=list(time="ms",
                        pinch="1", force="Newtons (Normalized)"))
```

In this example we first created the basis, and then used the
fFunction constructor to create the functional data object, onePinch.
The coefficients in onePinch are obtained as the least-squares fit or
projection of the function values (argument y) onto the space of the
basis functions. Notice that the function domain specified by the basis
must span the range of argument values. The argument fNames
associates character strings with functional data objects for labeling
purposes, for example, to give a name to the function or variable, to
name the units in the function argument, to name the values at which
the function is observed, or to name the units for the function values.

S+FDA includes a plot method for functional data objects. Here we
plot the onePinch object, and also include the observations in the plot
by a subsequent call to points (see Figure 3.1):

```
#Plot the fFunction object
> plot(onePinch, main="Pinch #1")
```

```
> points(pinchtime, pinchmat[, 1])
```

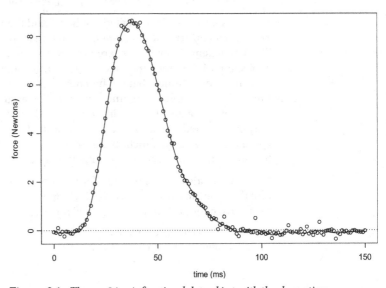

Pinch #1

Figure 3.1: *The onePinch functional data object with the observations superimposed.*

Notice that the function names from argument fNames in the constructor are used for labeling the plot.

Constructing from coefficients and a basis

You may construct an S+FDA object of class fFunction from an object of class fBasis, together with a vector of coefficients β_j. This method of construction is primarily used internally, but users may also have occasion to use it, for example, in simulation. Here we simulate a functional data object with noise added to the coefficients of onePinch:

```
> coef <- getCoef(onePinch)
> coef <- coef + rnorm(length(coef)) # add noise
> onePinch2 <- fFunction(coef, basis,
                    fNames=list(time="ms", pinch="1",
                    force="Newtons(Normalized)"))
```

The function getCoef is used to access the coefficients in onePinch.

Constructing from fFunction object or fVector object with length of I

It is also possible to create a smoother fFunction object from an existing fFunction object. See Chapter 4.

For an object of class fVector with length of 1, i.e., only one function in the vector, its class can be changed to fFunction. See example in later of this section.

Operations on Univariate Functional Data Objects

Once created, you may apply various operations to functional data objects. Smoothing is fundamental in functional data analysis, and is treated separately in Chapter 4. Below we discuss other important operations: evaluation, derivatives, inner products, and integrals for function objects.

Evaluation

Use the function fEval to evaluate a function, its derivatives with a linear differential operator applied to the function specified by the argument linDop, at arbitrary argument values within the domain of the function. Here, we evaluate the onePinch object at some arbitrary times.

```
> newtimes <- seq(1.5, 140.5, length=140)
> onePinchEval <- fEval(onePinch, fArg=newtimes)
```

Derivatives

Obtain derivatives of functional data objects using the constructing function in S+FDA. The following examples show how to compute and plot the first and second derivatives of the pinch force object, onePinch:

```
> onePinchEval1 <- fEval(onePinch, fArg=newtimes,
                                linDop=fDop(1))
> onePinchEval2 <- fEval(onePinch, fArg=newtimes,
                                linDop=fDop(2))
> par(mfrow=c(2,1))
> plot(fFunction(onePinch, linDop=fDop(1)),
        main="First Derivative")
> plot(fFunction(onePinch, linDop=fDop(2)),
        main="Second Derivative")
```

The resulting plot is given in Figure 3.2.

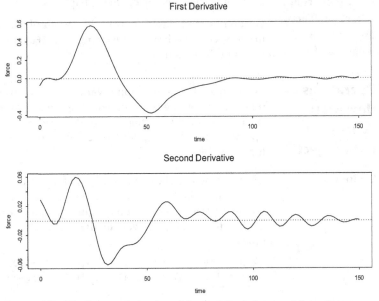

Figure 3.2: *The first two derivatives of the onePinch functional data object.*

The oscillations in the second derivative indicate that additional smoothing may be desirable.

Linear Differential Operator

We can also apply a linear differential operator to an fFunction object by specifying the argument linDop in the constructing function.

Here is an example:

```
> x <- seq(0,365)
> y <- sin(2*pi*x/365) + cos(4*pi*x/265)
> basis1 <- FourierBasis(c(0,365), nbasis=8)
> fun1 <- fFunction(basis1, y, x)
> fLinOp <- fVector(matrix(c(2,1),1,2),
                      constantBasis(c(0,365)))
> ex2 <- fFunction(fun1, linDop=fLinDopN(fLinOp))
```

where fLinOp is an object of class fVector having two fFunction
objects (see its definition in the next of this section) as the nonlinear
coefficients of the 0th and 1st derivatives in the linear differential
operator, and fLinDopN is the constructing function to create an object
of class fLinDopN for normalized linear differential operator. See
Chapter 4, or the help files of fFunction and fLinDopN, for more
detailed information about the definition of the linear differential
operator.

Integration

It is also possible to integrate functions (or linear differential operators
applied to a function) over an interval in the domain of the function
using the function fInt. Noting that the integral of the function
computed over any time interval gives the total exertion over that
interval, we compute the total exertion over the first 50 standardized
time units, and compare it with the total exertion for the curve:

```
> fInt(onePinch, limits=c(0,50))/fInt(onePinch)
```

The result indicates that 76.6 percent of the total exertion occurred in
the first 50 standardized time units.

A common use for integrals of positive functions is to standardize the
function so that its integral has the value 1, for example:

```
> onePinchStd <- onePinch/fInt(onePinch)
```

S+FDA provides another function, fIntExp, that integrates the
exponential of a function. It is useful for monotonic functional
smoothing since the resulting integral is monotonic (see the chapter
on smoothing), as well as for density estimation.

Inner Products

Inner products can be computed in S+FDA via the function fInProd.
The inner product of two functional data objects defined on the same
domain is the integral of their product over that domain. For
example, we can compute the inner product of the onePinch object
and its the first derivative as follows:

```
> fInProd(onePinch, fFunction(onePinch, linDop=fDop(1))))
```

or, equivalently,

```
> fInProd(onePinch, onePinch, linDop2=fDop(1))
```

Inner products can also be used to standardize the integrals of the
squared function values, for example:

```
> onePinchStd2 <- onePinch/sqrt(fInProd(onePinch))
```

Centering

The mean of a functional data object can be obtained by dividing the integral of the function by the length of its domain. Centering is possible by subtracting the mean from the function. The integral of the centered function vanishes. The resulting function can be further scaled by dividing by the integral, giving unit area under the absolute curve. These operations are accomplished as follows:

```
> onePinchInt <- fInt(onePinch)
> onePinchCtr <- (onePinch - onePinchInt/150)/onePinchInt
```

(150 is the length of the domain of the function).

Arithmetic Operators

It is also possible to apply the operators "+", "-", "*", "/", "sqrt", "^" to the functions (the exponentiation operator, "^" is restricted to constant values). As an example, we construct a polygonal basis for pinch force data:

```
> basis <- polygonalBasis(pinchtime)
> onePinchPolyg <- fFunction(basis, y=pinchmat[,1],
                                 fArgs=pinchtime)
```

and plot of the difference between onePinchPolyg and onePinch (with B-spline basis):

```
> par(mfrow=c(1,1))
> plot(onePinch - onePinchPolyg)
```

The result is shown in Figure 3.3.

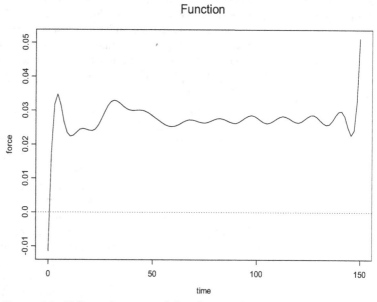

Figure 3.3: *Difference between pinch force function objects created with a B-spline and a polygonal basis.*

The differences between the two functions are small relative to the observed function values, which have a maximum magnitude near 8.

Vectors of Functional Data Objects

An object of class fFunction is the functional equivalent of a scalar. Vectors of functional data objects, each having the same basis, are represented by objects of class fVector. We will often refer to fVector objects as *variables,* since these are usually (but not always) observed as a quantity measured over a random sample, such as pinch force measured over a random sample of subjects. In addition to vectorized counterparts of operations on objects of class fFunction, it is also possible to form mean and variance functions for vectors of functional data objects.

Similar to fFunction objects, the operations of evaluation, derivatives, integrals, linear differential operator and inner products can be applied to an fVector objects.

Creating vectors of functional data objects

Construction of objects of class fVector is similar to that of objects of class fFunction. Instead of a vector of function values, the required input is a matrix of function values, in which each column corresponds to a separate function. Observations in a column that are missing are omitted in computations. This has no effect on the computations in other columns. Here we create an fVector using a polygonal basis from all twenty columns in the pinch force data described above:

```
> par(mfrow=c(2,1))
> basis <- polygonalBasis(pinchtime)
> pinchVecPolyg <- fVector(basis, y=pinchmat,
                           fArgs=pinchtime,
                           fNames=list(time="ms",
                           pinchForce=paste(1:20),
                           force="Newtons (Normalized)"))
> plot(pinchVecPolyg, main="Vector of Functions")
> basis <- bsplineBasis(range(pinchtime))
> pinchVecBspln <- fVector(basis, y=pinchmat,
                           fArgs=pinchtime,
                           fNames=list(time="ms",
                           pinchForce=paste(1:20),
                           force="Newtons (Normalized)"))
> plot(pinchVecBspln, main="Vector of Functions")
```

The result is displayed in Figure 3.4.

For an object of fVector with length of 1, it can be changed to an object of class fFunction. For example:

```
> pinchVecPolyg1 <- fFunction(pinchVecPolyg[1])
```

turns pinchVecPolyg1 to be an object of class fFunction.

Indexing

Objects of class fVector can be indexed in the same manner as a numeric vector. An fVector object is returned even when that fVector would be of length 1.

Sum of a vector of functions

The sum of an object of class fVector is an object of class fFunction representing the (point wise) sum function. For example:

```
> sumOnePinch <- sum(pinchVecPolyg)
```

Mean of a vector of functions

The mean of an object of class fVector is an object of class fFunction representing the (point wise) mean function. As an example, we compute and plot the vector of functions created from the pinch force data with a polygonal basis:

```
> plot(mean(pinchVecPolyg))
```

The result appears in the top half of Figure 3.5. Standardization of vector of functions to a point wise mean of zero is accomplished using intuitive operations:

```
> cntrPinchVec <- pinchVecPolyg - mean(pinchVecPolyg)
> plot(cntrPinchVec, main="Deviations from the mean")
```

The result is given in the bottom half of Figure 3.5.

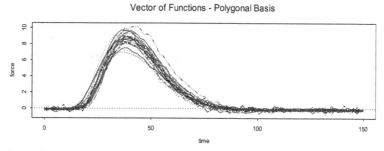

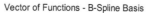

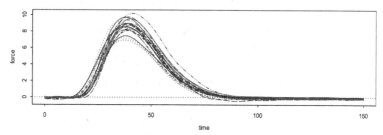

Figure 3.4: *Vectors of pinch force functions created with different bases.*

Variances

Pointwise variances (variances at each point in the domain) can also be computed in S+FDA via the function fVar. As an example, we compute and plot pointwise variances for the vectors of functions created from the pinch force data with the polygonal basis:

```
> varPinchVec <- fVar(pinchVecPolyg, bivariate=F)
> plot(varPinchVec, main="Pointwise Variances")
```

The result is displayed in the top part of Figure 3.6:.

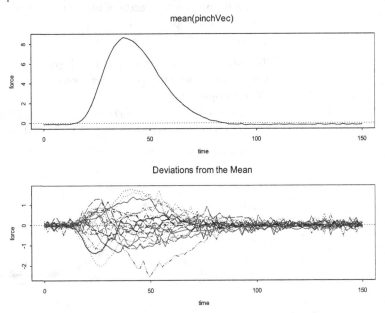

Figure 3.5: *Mean of the pinch force functions (top half). Pinch force functions standardized to a point wise mean of zero (bottom half).*

It is also possible to compute covariances between two vectors of values that are the results of evaluating an fVector object at two argument values. For example, let

```
> x1 <- fEval(pinchVecPolyg, 50)
> x2 <- fEval(pinchVecPolyg, 55)
```

Then the covariance between the functions at argument values 50 and 55 can be computed as follows:

```
> var(t(x1),t(x2))
```

This value turns out to be 0.827.

Generalizing this to all values in the domain of the function, a bivariate variance-covariance function can be defined by considering the covariance at any two arguments. The following example computes and plots this function for the polygonal basis representation of the pinch force data:

```
> covPinchVec <- fVar(pinchVecPolyg)
> plot(covPinchVec)
```

The plot is given in the bottom half of Figure 3.6:

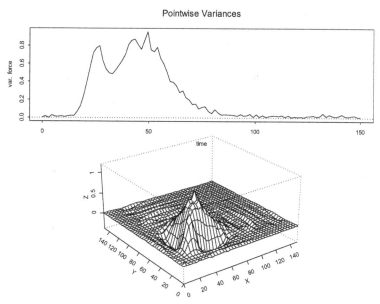

Figure 3.6: *The variance function (top), and the estimated variance-covariance function (bottom) for the pinch force functional data object.*

The following code can be used to verify that the covariance has the same value (0.827) at $50, 55$:

```
> fEval(covPinchVec, 50, 55)
```

List of Functional Data Objects

A list of functional data objects with possible different basis functions are represented by objects of class fList. The components of the fList object are objects of class fFunction.

Creating list of functional data objects

We can construct an fList object from objects of class fFunction, fVector, list, or fList.

Here is an example of creating an fList object from two fFunction objects:

```
> fBasis1 <- FourierBasis(c(0,365), nbasis=101)
```

59

```
> fBasis2 <- bsplineBasis(c(0, 365), nbasis=101)
> temp1 <- fFunction(fBasis1, tempav[,1], 1:365)
> prec1 <- fFunction(fBasis2, precav[,1], 1:365)
> fL1 <- fList(temp1, prec1)
```

Or, create an fList object from an fVector object:

```
> temp23 <- fVector(fBasis1, tempav[,2:3], 1:365)
> fL2 <- fList(temp23)
```

Or, create an fList object from a simple list of fFunction objects:

```
> fL3 <- fList(list(temp1, prec1))
```

Or, create an fList object from fList objects:

```
> fL4 <- fList(fL1, fL2)
```

Operations on fList Objects

Since any fList object is a list of fFunction objects, perform any operation by doing an lapply.

For example, to take the square root of fL4:

```
> lapply(fL4, sqrt)
```

BIVARIATE FUNCTIONAL DATA OBJECTS (EXAMPLE)

In this section we first describe the various constructors associated with bivariate functional data objects in S+FDA, and then discuss some of the most useful operations associated with these objects.

Constructing Bivariate Functional Data Objects

There are two possible bivariate functional data objects: fProdFunction and fFinElemFunction. Construct these using the corresponding constructors.

Construct a class fProdFunction object using the constructor in one of two ways:

- from data -- i.e., a vector of known function values, the matrix of arguments at which the functions are evaluated -- and a basis,

- from known bases coefficients and the corresponding bases.

from known basis coefficients and the two univariate bases. Construct fFinElemFunction objects from data -- i.e., a vector of known function values, the matrix of arguments at which the functions are evaluated -- and a basis, or from an fFinElemFunction existing object.

There are also functions for fitting linear models which return an object, one of whose components is a bivariate functional data object. This is discussed in greater detail in Chapter 6.

The constructor methods are now discussed in more detail.

Constructing from data and a basis

You may construct a bivariate function data object of either class fProdFunction or fFinElemFunction. We discuss each of these in turn.

As an example, we again consider the pinchmat dataset (see section Constructing Univariate Functional Data Objects on page 48). This time we model the variance-covariance surface.

First calculate the correlation of the data set pinchmat evaluated at the grid of (x, y) points, where x and y both range over 1:20.

```
> corPinch <- cor(pinchmat)
```

Construct a fProdFunction object by inputting an object of class fProdBasis, together with a matrix of known function values (observations) and two vectors for the arguments.

The first step is to create the fProdFunction object by first creating each of the component univariate bases. In this example, construct B-Spline and Fourier bases:

```
> fBasis1 <- bsplineBasis(c(1,20), nbasis=15, norder=2)
> fBasis2 <- FourierBasis(c(1,20), nbasis=15)
```

Next, construct the fProdFunction object

```
> fcorPinch1 <- fProdFunction(fProdBasis(fBasis1, fBasis2),
                              fVar=corPinch,
                              fArg1=1:20, fArg2=1:20,
                              bFNames=namesfcorPinch)
```

where

```
> namesfcorPinch <- list(args=list(arg1="Pinch",
                                    arg2="Pinch"),
                         vars="cor(Pinch)")
```

which gives names used in plot and print methods.

Alternatively, construct a fFinElemFunction object by inputting an object of class fFinElemBasis, together with a matrix of known function values and the two vectors of points at which the function are evaluated.

Create the finite element basis functions:

```
> fBasisFE <- fFinElemBasis(xDomain=c(1,20),
                            yDomain=c(1,20), params=c(19,19))
```

Given the basis functions fBasisFE, the data corPinch and $1:20$ for x and y, create an object of class fFinElemFunction by

```
> fcorPinchFE <- fFinElemFunction(fBasisFE,
                                  fVar=corPinch,
                                  fArg1=1:20, fArg2=1:20,
                                  bFNames=namesfcorPinch)
```

First, generate the graph of the original data set

```
> par(mfrow=c(1,1))
> persp(1:20, 1:20, corPinch)
```

The plot of `corPinch` is shown in Figure 3.7:

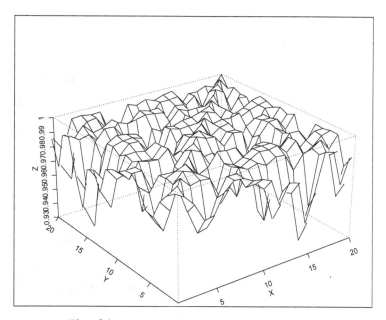

Figure 3.7: *Plot of the* `corPinch` *data.*

Next, compare the functional data objects created using the product basis and the finite element basis:

```
> par(mfrow=c(2,1))
> plot(fcorPinchProd)
> plot(fcorPinchFE)
```

The results are given in Figure 3.8:

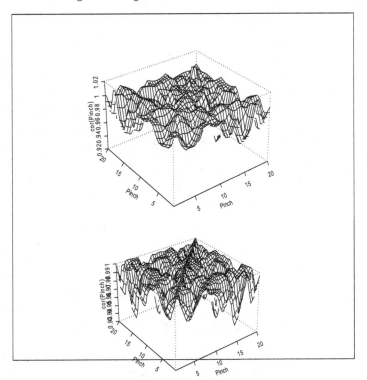

Figure 3.8: *Plots of the functional data objects for the* corPinch *data The top plot shows the FDA object constructed from a product basis, and the bottom shows that constructed from a finite element basis*

Note that it is also possible to have arbitrary evaluation points in constructing a fFinElemFunction object. In other words, the y values need not correspond to the same x's.

In this case, the arguments to the constructor function are a *vector* of known function values (observations) and a *matrix* of points at which the function is evaluated. See the help file for the fFinElemFunction constructor function for more details.

Constructing from coefficients and two univariate bases

You may construct an S+FDA object of class fProdFunction from two univariate objects of class fBasis, together with a matrix of coefficients β_{ij}. This method of construction is primarily used internally, but users may also have occasion to use it, for example, in simulation. Here we simulate a functional data object with noise added to the coefficients of fcorPinchProd:

```
> coef <- getCoef(fcorPinchProd)
> noise <- matrix(rnorm(nrow(coef)*ncol(coef)),
                      nrow=nrow(coef))
> coef <- coef + noise %*% t(noise)
> fcorPinchProd2 <- fProdFunction(coef, fBasis1, fBasis2)
```

The function getCoef is used to access the coefficients in fcorPinchProd.

Constructing from existing object

It is also possible to create a smoother fProdFunction or fFinElemFunction object from an existing object with the same class. See Chapter 4.

Operations on Bivariate Functional Data Objects

Once created, you may apply various operations to bivariate functional data objects: evaluate functions, derivatives, and integrals.

Evaluation

Use the function fEval to evaluate a function, or its derivatives at argument values within the domain of the function.

Suppose you want to evaluate the functional data objects at the following data points:

```
> x1 <- y1 <- seq(1.01, 19.9, length=20)
```

For easy comparison, create a two column matrix of the function evaluations. The first column contains the result from the product basis, the second for the finite element basis.

```
# evaluate
> fcorPinch.x1y1 <- cbind(as.vector(fEval(fcorPinchProd,
                           x1, y1)), fEval(fcorPinchFE, x1, y1))
```

The following code plots the results shown in Figure 3.9:

```
> par(mfrow=c(2,1))
```

```
> zlim <- range(fcorPinch.x1y1)
> persp(x1, y1, matrix(fcorPinch.x1y1[, 1],
                        ncol=length(x1)), zlim=zlim)
> persp(x1, y1, matrix(fcorPinch.x1y1[, 2],
                        ncol=length(x1)), zlim=zlim)
```

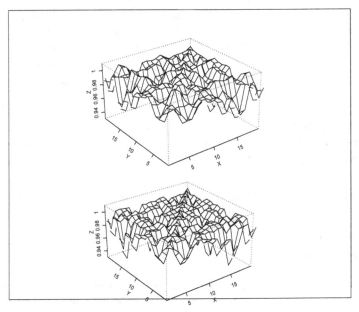

Figure 3.9: *Plots comparing function evaluations. The top plot is for the product basis, and the bottom is for the finite element basis.*

Derivatives

Obtain derivatives of functional data objects using the function fEval in S+FDA. The following example shows how to compute and plot the partial derivatives of the covariance matrix of pinchMat.

For easy comparison, create a two column matrix of the derivatives. The first column contains the result from the product basis, the second for the finite element basis.

```
> dxfcorPinch <- cbind(as.vector(fEval(fcorPinchProd, x1,
                        y1, linDop1=fDop(1))),
                        fEval(fcorPinchFE, x1, y1, xDeriv=1))
```

```
> dyfcorPinch <- cbind(as.vector(fEval(fcorPinchProd, x1,
                       y1, linDop2=fDop(1))),
                       fEval(fcorPinchFE, x1, y1, yDeriv=1))
```

The following code plots the results shown in Figure 3.10: for the derivative with respect to the first argument.

```
> zlim <- range(dxfcorPinch)
> persp(x1, y1, matrix(dxfcorPinch[,1], ncol=length(x1)),
        zlim=zlim)
```

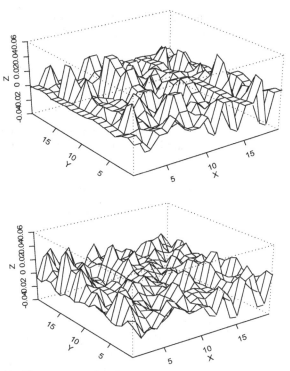

Figure 3.10: *Plots comparing first derivatives with respect to the first argument. The top plot is for the product basis, and the bottom is for the finite element basis.*

```
> persp(x1, y1, matrix(dxfcorPinch[, 2], ncol=length(x1)),
        zlim=zlim)
```

Integration   It is also possible to integrate functions over a region in the domain of
the function using fInt.   This is only possible for functions created
from a finite element basis.

$$\int\limits_{x_1 y_1(x)}^{x_2 y_2(x)} \int f(x, y)\,dx\,dy$$

Note that the lower and upper limits for the second argument may be
a function of the first argument.

As a simple example, integrate the functional data object of the
corPinch data, created from the finite element basis. By default the
region of integration is the entire domain.

```
> int.corPinch <- fInt(fcorPinchFE, eps=0.1)
```

In the next example, we integrate a plane, and integrate over limits
which are linear functions of the first argument. Specifically, we
integrate:

$$\int\limits_{0}^{10} \int\limits_{0.3x}^{0.3x + 3} (x + y)\,dx\,dy$$

To integrate over the desired limits, first calculate quantities that
define the domain. Integrate x from 0 to 10, and y from limits that
are linear functions of x.

```
> xUpperLimit <- 10
> slope <- 0.3
> intercept <- 3
> n <- 11      # number of points for x domain
> x <- seq(0, xUpperLimit, len=n) # x domain
> yLowerLimit <- slope*x
```

```
> yUpperLimit <- slope*x + intercept
```

Next create functional data objects for the limits of integration, $y_1(x)$ and $y_2(x)$

```
> fBasis1 <- bsplineBasis(c(0, xUpperLimit), nbasis=n,
                          norder=2)
> fyLower <- fFunction(fBasis1, yLowerLimit, x)
> fyUpper <- fFunction(fBasis1, yUpperLimit, x)
```

Then create a functional data object for the integrand,

```
> z <- matrix(nrow=n, ncol=n)
> for(i in x) z[i+1, ] <- i+x
> fBasisFE <- fFinElemBasis(c(0,xUpperLimit),
                            c(0,xUpperLimit), params=c(4,4))
> fun <- fFinElemFunction(fBasisFE, fVal=z, fArg1=x)
```

Finally, integrate:

```
> int.fun <- fInt(fun, lowArg1=0, upArg1=xUpperLimit,
                  lowArg2=fyLower, upArg2=fyUpper)
```

The exact answer can be calculated as:

```
> exactAnswer <-0.5*intercept*xUpperLimit*(xUpperLimit
                + slope*xUpperLimit + intercept)
> c(int.fun, exactAnswer )
[1] 240 240
```

which agrees.

LINEAR DIFFERENTIAL OPERATORS AND SMOOTHING

4

LINEAR DIFFERENTIAL OPERATORS

Linear differential operators are used extensively throughout the S+FDA library. These operators can be applied to functions and evaluated, or used as smoothing penalty functions.

Perhaps the simplest linear differential operators are derivative operators of any given order (including order 0, which gives the function itself). The general form of a linear differential operator is:

$$Lf(t) = \sum_{k=0}^{m-1} w_k(t)D^k f(t) + D^m f(t)$$

where $D^k f(t)$ denotes the kth derivative of $f(t)$ with respect to t, (D^k is a derivative operator), and the $w_k(t)$ are specified objects of class fFunction.

In S+FDA, linear differential operators are specified as objects of class fLinDop, which includes subclasses fLinDopN for normalized linear differential operators (weight function for highest-order derivative is the constant 1) and fDop for simple derivative operators. For example, fDop(2) denotes the second-derivative operator.

SMOOTHING VIA A ROUGHNESS PENALTY

Smoothing when Constructing Functional Data Objects

Bases computed using least-squares methods may result in fits that are highly oscillatory - especially when many basis functions are used. To avoid such overfitting, roughness penalties may be added to the least-squares criterion when constructing functional data objects from observed data. S+FDA provides the option of specifying a penalty term for creating smoothed functional data objects using the roughness penalty approach. In constructing a smoothed function from observed data, the penalized least-squares criterion has the following form:

- for univariate functional data:

$$\phi_\lambda(\beta) = \sum_{i=1}^{n} \left(y_i - \sum_{j=1}^{n_b} \beta_j b_j(x_i) \right)^2 + \lambda \int_T \left\{ L \left[\sum_{j=1}^{n_b} \beta_j b_j(x) \right] \right\}^2 dx :$$

- for bivariate functional data with product basis functions:

$$\phi_\lambda(\beta) = \sum_{k=1}^{n} \left(z_k - \sum_{i=1}^{n_x} \sum_{j=1}^{n_y} \beta_{ij} b_i^x(x_k) b_j^y(y_k) \right)^2 +$$

$$\lambda \cdot \int_{T_x} \int_{T_y} \left\{ \sum_{i=1}^{n_x} \sum_{j=1}^{n_y} L[b_i^x(x)] \beta_{ij} L[b_j^y(y)] \right\}^2 dx dy$$

- for bivariate functional data with linear finite element basis functions:

$$\phi_\lambda(\beta) = \sum_{k=1}^{n} \left[z_k - \sum_{j=1}^{n_b} \beta_j \Phi_j(x_k, y_k) \right]^2 +$$

$$\lambda \cdot \int\int_T \left\{ \sum_{j=1}^{n_b} \beta_j [\Phi_{j,x}(x,y) + \Phi_{j,y}(x,y)] \right\}^2 dx dy$$

where L is a *linear differential operator,* and λ is a penalty parameter that must be specified.

The goal is to estimate the functional coefficients β. You may use any linear combination of derivatives of the basis functions to specify the linear differential operator in the penalty term. A good rule of thumb is to include in the penalty a derivative of order two greater than the highest derivative of interest. This will penalize the curvature (second derivative) of the derivative of interest. Also make sure that the underlying basis is sufficiently smooth for the penalty to make sense.

The idea in a roughness penalty approach is to penalize *roughness,* as defined by the square of the given combination of derivatives in the final term of the above equation, so that the resulting function estimate (or its derivative) is smooth. The positive parameter λ specifies the amount of smoothing. Larger values give more weight to the penalty and thus increase the amount of smoothing.

Smoothing Functional Data Objects

You may also smooth functional data objects after they have been created. In this case, the criterion to be minimized is the sum of the (1) integrated squared distance between the smoothed and the unsmoothed function, plus (2) the penalty parameter as follows:

- for univariate functional data:

$$\phi_\lambda(\beta) = \int \left[f(x) - \sum_{j=1}^{n_b} \beta_j b_j(x) \right]^2 dx + \lambda \int \left\{ L\left[\sum_{j=1}^{n_b} \beta_j b_j(x) \right] \right\}^2 dx$$

- for bivariate functional data with product basis functions:

$$\phi_\lambda(\beta) = \int\int \left(f(x,y) - \sum_{i=1}^{n_x} \sum_{j=1}^{n_y} \beta_{ij} b_i^x(x) b_j^y(y) \right)^2 dx dy +$$

$$\lambda \cdot \int_{T_x} \int_{T_y} \left\{ \sum_{i=1}^{n_x} \sum_{j=1}^{n_y} L[b_i^x(x)] \beta_{ij} L[b_j^y(y)] \right\}^2 dx dy$$

- for bivariate functional data with linear finite element basis functions:

$$\phi_\lambda(\beta) = \iint \left[f(x,y) - \sum_{j=1}^{n_b} \beta_j \Phi_j(x,y) \right]^2 dxdy +$$

$$\lambda \cdot \iint_T \left\{ \sum_{j=1}^{n_b} \beta_j [\Phi_{j,x}(x,y) + \Phi_{j,y}(x,y)] \right\}^2 dxdy$$

Again the goal is to estimate the functional coefficients β_j or β_{ij}, but here the functions $f(x)$, or $f(x,y)$, are "known" functions that have already been expressed as a basis functions expansion:

$$f(x) = \Sigma \beta_j \tilde{b}_j(x),$$

or

$$f(x,y) = \Sigma\Sigma \beta_{ij} \tilde{b}_i^x(x) \tilde{b}_j^y(y)$$

or

$$f(x,y) = \Sigma \beta_i \tilde{\Phi}_i(x,y) .$$

When to Smooth?

It is important to note that the two smoothing techniques (smoothing from the observed data, or smoothing an existing function) can lead to different results, and different values of the smoothing parameter λ may be desired. The smoothing process is exploratory in nature and cannot be automated to accommodate all problems of interest.

Oversmoothing when creating the functional data object, or at any point in a sequence of functional data operations, can result in loss of information. In general, in order to retain maximal information, it is safer to smooth only when necessary. Regularization should be deferred as much as possible to the final functional data object to be estimated (e.g. functional regression coefficients or principal components).

Pinch Force Data Example for Univariate Functional Data

The functional data object onePinchBspln constructed from the pinch force data using a B-spline basis expansion in Chapter 3 is already somewhat smooth because of:

- the choice of cubic splines for the basis, and

- the relatively limited number of basis functions (23) used in fitting the functions to the 151 observed data points.

By contrast, the functional data object for the pinch force data constructed from a polygonal basis in Chapter 3 (onePinchPolyg) is a good candidate for smoothing techniques since it contains the observations joined by line segments.

Create the functional data object from observed data and the polygonal bases constructed from the observation times:

```
> onePinchPolyg <- fFunction(polygonalBasis(pinchtime),
                           y=pinchmat[, 1], fArgs=pinchtime)
```

Next, apply a smoothing operation to create a smoothed object, in this case by penalizing the first derivative:

```
> pinchSmooth2 <- fFunction(onePinchPolyg,
                    penalty=list(lambda=100,linDop=fDop(2)),
                    basis=bsplineBasis(range(pinchtime),
                        norder=3,
                        breaks=seq(pinchtime[1],
                               pinchtime[length(pinchtime)],
                               length=50)))
```

Note that we specify a new basis for the smoothed object. The original basis does not have a sufficient number of derivatives for the specified penalty term to be nonzero. Generally, if the basis for the functional data object is sufficiently smooth, you may construct a smoothed object directly from the basis and the observed data.

Correlation of Pinch Force Data Example for Bivariate Functional Data

A two dimensional example is given by the data corPinch, the correlation of the data set pinchmat, created in Chapter 3. We construct a smoothed functional data object first using the product basis, then the finite element basis.

To construct a basis function object of class fProdBasis, first create each of the component univariate bases. In this example, construct B-Spline and Fourier bases:

```
> fBasis1 <- bsplineBasis(c(1,20), nbasis=15, norder=2)
> fBasis2 <- FourierBasis(c(1,20), nbasis=15)
> fBasis12 <- fProdBasis(fBasis1, fBasis2)
```

Create the bivariate functional data object from the function values and variables:

```
> fcorPinch <- fProdFunction(fBasis12, fVar=corPinch,
                              fArg1=1:20)
```

Create the smoothed bivariate functional data object by penalizing the first derivatives on both arguments of the function:

```
> fcorPinchSm <- fProdFunction(fBasis12, fVar=corPinch,
                 fArg1=1:20, penalty=list(lambda=1000,
                 linDop1=fDop(1), linDop2=fDop(1)))
```

Next, create the bivariate functional data with basis function of class fFinElemBasis.

```
> fBasis <- fFinElemBasis(xDomain=c(1,20), yDomain=c(1,20),
                          params=c(19, 19))
> fcorPinch2 <- fFinElemFunction(object=fBasis,
                                 fVar=as.vector(corPinch),
                                 fArg1=cbind(rep(1:20, length=20),
                                             rep(1:20, each=20)))
```

and the smoothed functional data object:

```
> fcorPinchSm2 <- fFinElemFunction(object=fBasis,
                                   fVar=as.vector(corPinch),
                                   fArg1=cbind(rep(1:20, length=20),
                                               rep(1:20, each=20)),
                                   lambda=0.5)
```

We plot the smoothed functional data with two different basis functions as follows:

```
> par(mfrow=c(2, 1))
> plot(fcorPinchSm)
```

```
> plot(fcorPinchSm2)
```

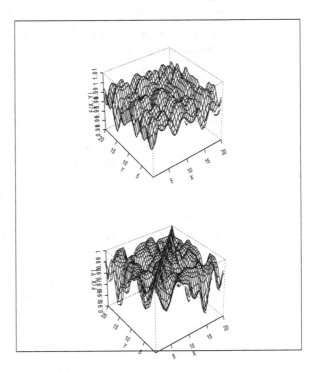

Figure 4.1: *The top plot is the smoothed functional data object with product basis functions and the bottom one is the smoothed functional data with finite element basis functions..*

SPECIFYING THE PENALTY FUNCTION

Smooth a functional data object by specifying the functional form of the smoothing term, via the penalty argument in functional data object constructors such as fFunction or fVector. For example, the following second-order linear differential operator is a common choice:

$$Lb_j(x) = \frac{d^2 b_j(x)}{dx^2} = D^2 b_j(x)$$

In the above example we smoothed functional data that had a polygonal basis using this second-order penalty, but in order to do so we had to change the basis to one that is sufficiently smooth to have a nonzero penalty.

Below we plot the original function, its transformation onePinchBspln to a B-spline basis, and the smoothed function resulting from applying the roughness penalty with that same B-spline basis:

```
> onePinchSpln <- fFunction(bsplineBasis(range(pinchtime),
                    norder=4,
                    breaks=seq(pinchtime[1],
                      pinchtime[length(pinchtime)],
                      length=50)),
                    y=pinchmat[,1], fArgs=pinchtime)

> par(mfrow=c(2,1))
> plot(onePinchPolyg, lty=8,
       main="Function with Polygonal and B-Spline Bases")
> lines(onePinchSpln, lwd=2)
> plot(onePinchPolyg, lty=8,
       main="Polygonal Function and Second Order Smooth")
> lines(pinchSmooth2, lwd=2)
```

The results are displayed in Figure 4.2::

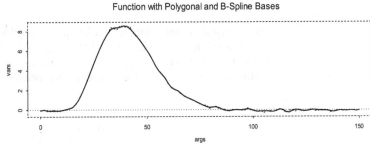

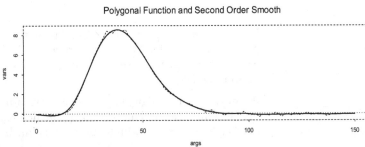

Figure 4.2: *The first instance of the pinch force data fit with polygonal and B-spline bases (top). The polygonal fit and fit obtained when smoothing with a second order roughness penalty (bottom). The functional data with polygonal basis is indicated by the dotted line in both cases.*

The results show that using the penalty produces a smoother function.

Height Data Example

In Chapter 1, we used a penalty on the second derivative to smooth a functional form of the height data. If we smooth with the same penalty parameter, 0.001, on the fourth derivative, we obtain a much smoother second derivative, although the oscillatory behavior of the function away from the endpoints indicates that further smoothing might be desirable (see Figure 4.3).

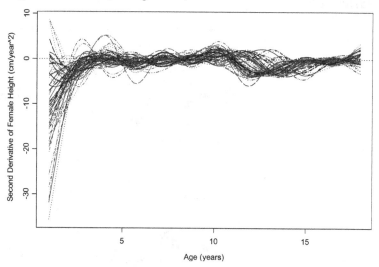

Figure 4.3: *Second derivatives of the functional representation of the female height data. The fourth derivative was penalized for smoothing, with penalty parameter 0.001.*

Effect of Penalty Parameter

As an example of the effect of the smoothing penalty parameter, we smooth the height data using a penalty on the fourth derivative for `lambda = 0.00002, 0.1. 0.5, 2.0`. Figure 4.3 shows the second derivative of female height for each of these values of `lambda`:

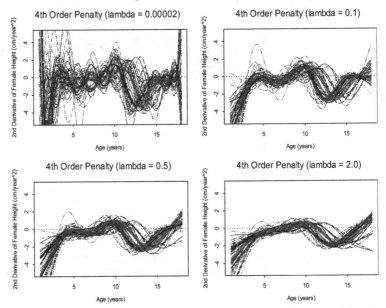

Figure 4.4: *Second derivative of the female height data when the functional data is formed using a 4th order penalty.*

As might be expected, the larger penalty parameter results in a significantly smoother second derivative.

Penalizing Linear Combinations of Derivatives

You may also smooth by using the square of a linear differential operator as the smoothing penalty. Specify this via the `linDop` component of the `penalty` argument to `fFunction` or `fVector`.

Generalized Cross Validation

The goal is to choose a `lambda` that minimizes errors when predicting new observations. If the errors for each `lambda` were known, it would be possible to plot the errors vs. `lambda`, and choose the `lambda` corresponding to the minimum error.

However, the errors are not known and so it is necessary to estimate the prediction error that would result from each lambda. The sum of squared residuals gives an optimistic estimate of error because the same data is used to both fit the model, and assess its performance.

Leave-one-out cross-validation calculates n fits. For $i = 1, \ldots n$:

- omit data point i, and estimate the smoothed function from the remaining data,
- predict the omitted case, and
- calculate the *deleted residual,* which is the difference between the observed response and the prediction.

The sum of squares of these deleted residuals honestly estimates the prediction error.

However, cross-validation has two problems (Ramsay and Silverman, 2004). First, it is computationally expensive, especially for large n. Second, it tends to undersmooth the data, tending to choose a lambda that results in fitting noisy variation that should be ignored.

Generalized cross validation (GCV) is a modified form of cross validation which avoids the computational expense of cross validation. It also tends to avoid undersmoothing. Please see Craven and Wahba (1979) or Green and Silverman (1994) for details. In brief, the deleted residuals can be obtained from the ordinary residuals by dividing by a factor. GCV replaces these individual factors by their average value, or *equivalent degrees of freedom.*

For the height data example in Chapter 1, the smooth was defined by a penalty on the second derivatives, and the value of lambda used was actually the optimal cross validated penalty parameter. Below we illustrate how we chose this value, by computing the smooth for a number of values of lambda. The values shown here are in an interval (determined by trial and error) that contains a local minimum:

```
> heightBasis
      <- bsplineBasis(fDomain=range(heightData$age),
                       nbasis=16, norder=6)
> lambda <- c(0.0001, 0.00025, 0.0005, 0.00075, 0.001,
              0.0015, 0.002, 0.0025)
> gcv <- numeric(length(lambda))
```

```
> for(i in 1:length(lambda))
      gcv[i] <- attributes(fVector(object=heightBasis,
                 y=heightData[,2:94], fArgs=heightData$age,
               · penalty=list(lambda=lambda[i],
                 linDop=fDop(2))))$gcv
```

A plot of the generalized cross validation statistic versus the logarithm of the penalty parameter can be created as follows (see Figure 4.5):

```
> par(mfrow=c(1,1))
> plot(log(lambda), gcv,
       ylab="Generalized cross validation")
> lines(log(lambda), gcv, lty=1)
```

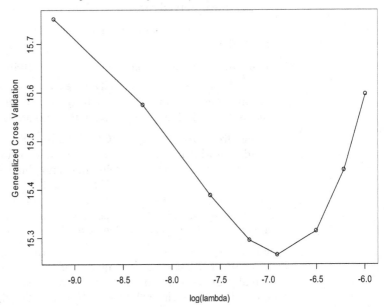

Figure 4.5: *Generalized cross validation statistic for the functional height data with penalized second derivative.*

The display shows that the optimal smoothing parameter corresponds to log(lambda) = -6.9 or lambda = 0.001, the value that was used to obtain the results in Chapter 1.

Trade-off Between Smoothing and Prediction

Prediction error is a measure of how well the resulting function predicts the observed data, rather than a measure of smoothness. To obtain smoother second derivatives for the height data than those obtained above and in Chapter 1, either use a larger penalty parameter or a different penalty function.

In the case of the height data, the rule of thumb suggests that a fourth-derivative penalty should be used to obtain smooth second derivatives. Yet using such a penalty with corresponding optimal cross validated penalty parameter (approximately 0.00002) yields a result whose second derivative is virtually identical to that obtained in Chapter 1.

The most practical approach is to examine the functional data and any derivatives of interest for a few choices of lambda, and choose one that has the desired smoothness properties while retaining reasonable predictive ability. Figure 4.6 shows the difference between predicted and observed values of female height for smoothing using a fourth order penalty for the same values of lambda used in Figure 4.3:

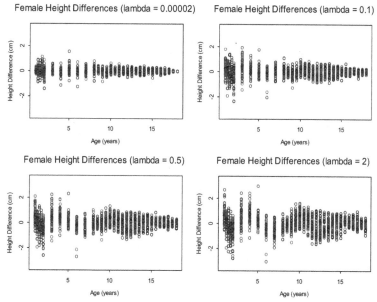

Figure 4.6: *Difference between predicted and observed female height for functional data formed using a fourth order smoothing penalty.*

85

As expected, the prediction ability decreases as the smoothing parameter is increased. The residuals are smallest for lambda = 0.00002, which is close to the optimal cross validated penalty parameter. Yet Figure 4.3 shows that the second derivative is highly oscillatory for this value of the penalty parameter. In this case the choice of lambda = 0.5 is probably a reasonable compromise between smoothness and prediction.

FUNCTIONAL REGISTRATION

5

Functional data analyses assume that a random sample of functions are comparable. Often this is not the case. For example, in the bone shape data discussed in more detail in the chapter on principal components, the shape of a bone surface is extracted from an x-ray of the bone by creating functions $x(d)$ and $y(d)$ that trace out an outline of the bone as a function of the distance traveled along the bone surface, d. The total distance traveled, the length of the bone surface, is adjusted to a distance of one, eliminating bone size from consideration, and making it possible to compare bone shapes through the functions $x(d)$ and $y(d)$. This is a simple example of *registration*, which is concerned with eliminating uninteresting differences in functions so that the remaining functional variation is (more) completely concerned with the differences of interest - in the bone data, we were concerned with bone shape, not bone size. Standardizing to a bone length of one does much to eliminate uninteresting variation in the bone curves, but it ignores differences that may be caused by different starting or ending positions on the bone surface, and differences due to bone orientation, e.g., angle of the leg bone on an x-ray. Ideally, these differences would also be eliminated or otherwise accounted for in a bone shape analysis, preferably using a model-based manner incorporating, say, shift and/ or scaling parameters. In practice, uninteresting differences in curves must often be eliminated in a more ad hoc fashion.

ANALYTIC REGISTRATION

Analytic methods may be used to register curves by optimizing a functional criterion. For each observation i, let $f_i(t)$ be either the functional data object or one of its derivatives, and let $g(t)$ be a target function (in the absence of other information, an estimate of the overall mean of the f_i). The basic idea behind the S+FDA function fRegister is to find a parameterized monotonic warping function $h_i(t, \gamma_i)$ for each function $f_i(t)$ such that $f_i(h_i(t, \gamma_i))$ closely matches the *target* function $g(t)$ in a penalized least squares sense. Here the γ_i are the parameters, and the penalized least-squares criterion is:

$$\phi(\gamma) = \sum_{i=1}^{n} \int [f_i(h_i(s, \gamma_i)) - g(s)]^2 ds + \lambda \int [h_i''(s, \gamma_i)]^2 ds$$

where the integrals are over the domain of the function. Notice that the penalty term which includes the penalty parameter λ is for smoothing the warping functions $h_i(t, \gamma_i)$.

Rather than registering the functions, it is also possible to register a linear combination of each functions and one or more of its derivatives. That is, it is also possible to register the results of applying a linear differential operator to the functions $f_i(t)$.

While any monotonic warping function h_i is possible, in S+FDA the parameters γ_i in the warping function define an intercept and slope, and also the coefficients of the basis functions of a class fFunction object. Specifically, the warping functions in fRegister have the following form:

$$h_i(t|c_{0i}, c_{1i}, \rho_i) = c_{0i} + c_{1i} \int_L^t \left(\exp \int_L^u w(v, \rho_i)dv \right) du$$

where L is the lower bound on the range of the function, u is the upper bound, and $w(v, \rho_i)$ is function represented by a B-spline basis. The parameters of each h_i include the slope c_{0i} and intercept c_{1i} as well as the coefficients and parameters (denoted by ρ_i)of the B-spline basis. Function fRegister has defaults for the knots and order of the B-splines, which can be chosen by users.

Although it is theoretically possible to optimize the criterion $\phi(\gamma)$ given above, in practice the problem becomes much more tractable if optimization is performed over a grid of points. This is what is done in fRegister. After estimating the warping functions h_i and obtaining the registered curves $f_i(h_i(s, \gamma_i))$ over a grid of points, the estimates are projected onto the basis used in the functions $f_i(t)$, and returned as the fWarp and fReg components of the output from fRegister. The details are given in Chapter 5 of Ramsay and Silverman (1997) and in the references cited there.

LIP MOTION EXAMPLE

Consider the measurement of the lower lip position as a single individuals says the syllable "bob" (see Ramsay and Silverman, 1997). Lower lip position was measured at 51 times for 20 replications over a (standardized) 650 millisecond interval. Measurements were made on a single individual. Time has already been registered to the same beginning and ending positions, with a standardized time length of 1. The data was fitted using an order 6 B-spline basis with 31 basis functions. No smoothing was performed. These operations are accomplished as follows:

```
> lipBasis <- fBasis(type="bspline", fDomain=c(0,1),
                     nbasis=31, params=(c(1:25)/26))
> fLip <- fVector(object=lipBasis, y=lipmat, fArgs=liptime,
                  fNames=list(NormalizedTime=liptime,
                  Replications=seq(20), Units="mm"))
```

The resulting functional data curves and their derivatives are displayed in Figure 5.1:

```
> par(mfrow=c(2,1))
> plot(fLip, main="Lower Lip Curves for \"bob\"")
> plot(fVector(fLip, linDop=fDop(1)),
       main="Derivative Lower Lip Curves for \"bob\"")
```

Although the 20 curves begin and end at the same locations after registration, some features (e.g., the point at which the curve minimum occurs) seem to be out of alignment. For example, in the plot of the first derivatives shown in the bottom of Figure 5.1, the shifts in extrema around 0.2 and 0.9 are particularly noticeable. Such differences may be important in an analysis.

We use the S+FDA function fRegister to register the first derivatives of the curves:

```
> regLip1 <- fRegister(fLip, mean(fLip), nDeriv=1,
                       maxIter=120, lambda=0.1,
                       criterion=1, penalty=0.0005)
```

The function fRegister requires a target function, taken here to be the derivative of the mean of the lip curves. Since this mean is itself a function of the curves we intend to register, additional calls to fRegister may improve the registration process:

```
> regLip1 <- fRegister(fLip, mean(regLip1$fReg),
                       nDeriv=1, maxIter=120, lambda=0.1,
                       criterion=1, penalty=0.0005)
```

The registered functions are contained in the fReg component of regLip1, and the target function in the second call to fRegister is the derivative of their mean.

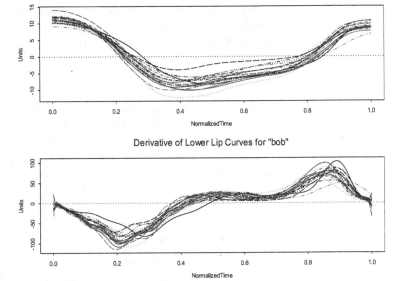

Figure 5.1: *Lower lip position during twenty utterances of the syllable "bob" (top) with derivatives (bottom).*

In the example call to fRegister we set nDeriv=1. This means that we are registering with respect to the first derivatives rather than the functions. We also provide two smoothing parameters, lambda, which is used in smoothing the warping functions, and penalty, which is used only when the warping function is based upon the derivatives (nDeriv > 0). In this case, the registered functions are estimated from the warping functions using smoothing splines with penalty parameter equal to penalty. It may take some experimentation with the lambda and penalty parameters to obtain satisfactory results.

The registered lip data is plotted as follows:

```
> par(mfrow=c(2,1))
```

```
> plot(regLip1$fReg,
        main="Registered Lower Lip Curves for \"bob\"")
> plot(fVector(regLip1$fReg, linDop=fDop(1)), main=
    "Derivative of Registered Lower Lip Curves for \"bob\"")
```

The results are given in Figure 5.2. Comparing with Figure 5.1, we see that both the functions and especially the derivatives are closer together, and that we no longer have large shifts in the derivative extrema. The estimates for the warping functions are given in Figure 5.3, in which we see that they are not strictly monotone due to round off errors.

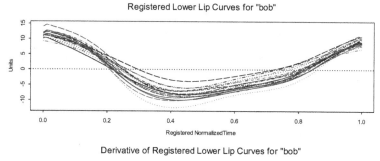

Registered Lower Lip Curves for "bob"

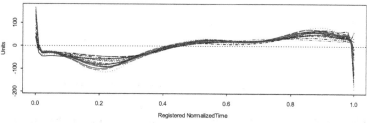

Derivative of Registered Lower Lip Curves for "bob"

Figure 5.2: *Registration for the lip data using function fRegister.*

Some cautions Analytic registration finds warping functions to minimize a least squares or similar criterion. One possible method for doing this is to make curve amplitudes as similar as possible. While the warping function does not modify the function values, warping simply to minimize amplitude (rather than features) can have significant impact on the curves - in trying to eliminate curve differences we may introduce artificial curve differences that can impact or even drive the results of any further analysis. As an example illustration of this problem, we use the fRegister function to register the lip data curves rather than their derivatives:

```
> regLip0 <- fRegister(fLip, mean(fLip), maxIter=100)
```

Both the registered and unregistered curves are shown in Figure 5.4. In this display we see that the registered curves are indeed very close together (minimizing the integrated squared distance), but that we have also introduced small artificial bumps near the minimum that are now the main feature differentiating the curves.

Lower Lip Curve Warping Functions

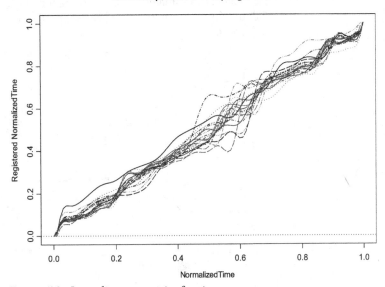

Figure 5.3: *Lower lip curve warping functions.*

Warping Functions

Warping functions are interesting in themselves because they contain information on how the curves were "aligned" in their arguments. This information is lost in the registered functions. If the warping function goes above/below the diagonal, the function is shifted in the positive/negative direction. These trends can be made more apparent in a plot that subtracts the diagonal from the warping curves. For the lip data, the warping functions contain information about how parts of the syllable are extended in length, while other parts are contracted, from one replication to the next.

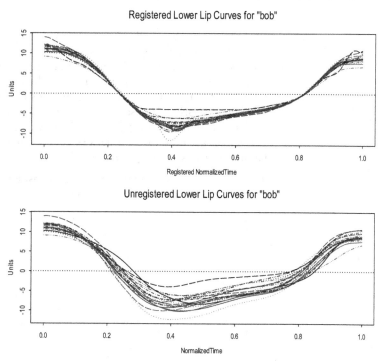

Figure 5.4: *Registered curves (top) and unregistered curves (bottom).*

LANDMARK REGISTRATION

Even though we generally have features or *landmarks* (e.g., extrema) in mind, the analytic registration used in function fRegister does not directly account for them. In landmark registration, the location of function landmarks are specified, often by hand, and a warping function is then obtained (by contracting or stretching the domain) so that all landmarks of the same type occur at the same position. Care must be taken in selecting the curve landmarks, especially if derivatives are used for landmark selection. Choosing the wrong landmarks can yield misleading results.

To see how landmarks might be defined, consider an enlarged version of the first derivatives for the lip data.

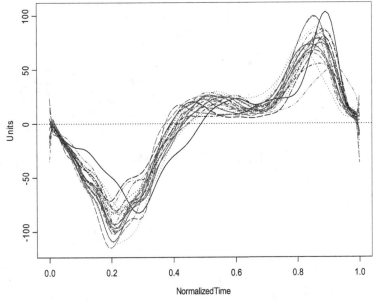

Figure 5.5: *First derivatives for the lip data.*

In the derivative curves, we chose four landmarks: 1) near time zero, some curves ascend before they descend. The first landmark is the position of the beginning of the descent near time zero. 2) The minimum around 0.2 is chosen for the second landmark. 3) the point at which the derivative curve crosses the horizontal axis is chosen as landmark 3. This is the location of the curve mimimum. 4) The maximum around 0.9 is the final landmark.

To find the horizontal location of these extrema, we first discretize the data, and then use the S-PLUS function identify as follows:

```
> nmarks <- 4
> x <- (1:200)/201
> lipmat <- fEval(fVector(fLip, linDop=fDop(1)), x)
> par(mfrow=c(1,1),pty='m')
> lipMarks <- matrix(0,20,nmarks)
> for (i in 1:20) {
     plot(x, lipmat[,i], main=paste('Curve',i))
     abline(h=0)
     index <- identify(x, lipmat[,i], n=nmarks)
     lipMarks[i,] <- x[index]
  }
```

Twenty curves are plotted, one at a time. For each curve, we use the mouse to identify the four landmarks. This yields a matrix, lipMarks, containing four columns and twenty rows, one for each of the 20 functions. Given the lipMarks matrix, landmark registration can then performed using the landmarkReg function as follows:

```
> landLip <- landmarkReg(fLip, mean(fLip), lipMarks)
```

Notice that although the landmarks were found using the derivative curve, the function curves are registered (rather than the derivatives).

The fReg and fWarp components of the landLip object contain the registered curves (here the first derivatives) and the warping functions, respectively. The registered curves are given in Figure 5.6, while the warping functions are given in Figure 5.7. In Figure 5.6, we see that the landmarks are indeed aligned along the horizontal axis.

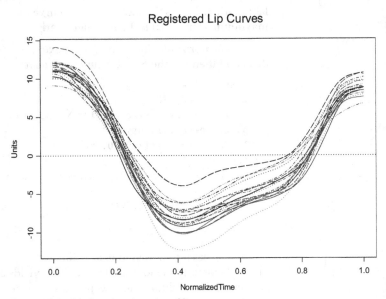

Figure 5.6: *Landmark registration of lip curves.*

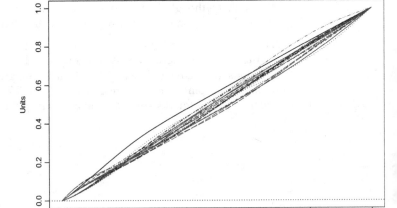

Figure 5.7: *Warping functions for landmark registration of the lip curves.*

Derivatives of registered curves
We now consider the derivatives of the registered curves, which can plotted by

```
> plot(fVector(landLip$fReg, linDop=fDop(1)))
```

which gives Figure 5.8.

Derivatives of Registered Lip Curves

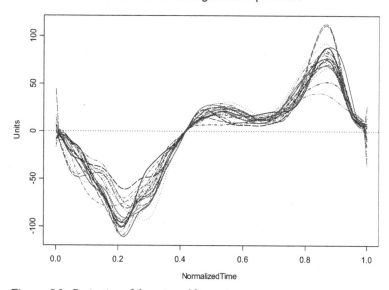

Figure 5.8: *Derivatives of the registered lip motion curves.*

The registered curves clearly show the effects of registration: the curves all cross the horizontal axis at the same point near 0.4, and the minimums around 0.2 and the maximums around 0.9 are aligned. There are also some undesirable effects, in particular the variation in the curves from 0 to 0.2.

Summary
In summary, the aim of registration is to align sets of functions so that comparison is possible at each argument value. Registration is often an unavoidable aspect of functional data analysis, but it can have unintended consequences, and must be applied with caution.

FUNCTIONAL LINEAR MODELS

6

Linear regression is one of the most commonly used methods in statistics. In linear regression the expected value of a dependent variable, y, is predicted using one or more independent variables or predictors, x. A least-squares criterion is minimized in fitting the model to obtain estimates. Often the interest is in simply in obtaining good predictors of the dependent variable, but linear regression models are also used to study relationships between variables. Functional linear models extend linear regression methods to allow functional independent and/or dependent variables.

We begin the chapter with a mathematical description of a functional linear model. This is followed by some examples.

Functional Dependent Variables

Perhaps the simplest functional linear model is one in which the dependent variable is a function, and the predictors or independent variables are scalar. In this case, at each point t in the function domain, estimates of the dependent variable can be obtained using a linear model in the predictors. Because the regression coefficients depend upon t, they too are functions of t. For example, a two predictor model would have the form

$$y(t) = \beta_0(t) + \beta_1(t)x_1 + \beta_2(t)x_2 + \varepsilon(t)$$

Here x_1 and x_2 are the two scalar predictors, $y(t)$ is the functional dependent variable, $\beta_0(t)$, $\beta_1(t)$, and $\beta_2(t)$ are coefficient functions, and $\varepsilon(t)$ is the error term. Clearly, for each $t = t_k$, estimates for $\beta_0(t_k)$, $\beta_1(t_k)$, and $\varepsilon(t_k)$ can be obtained by fitting a linear regression model.

Functional Independent Variables

Now consider the case in which the dependent variable is scalar, but the independent variables are functions. The model takes the form

$$y = \beta_0 + \int (\beta_1(s)x_1(s) + \beta_2(s)x_2(s))ds + \varepsilon$$

This model has two functional predictors, $x_1(s)$ and $x_2(s)$, with two coefficient functions, $\beta_1(s)$ and $\beta_2(s)$, an intercept coefficient, β_0, and an error ε. Because the independent variables and associated coefficients are functional, we integrate over their values to obtain the contribution of the independent variable. Methods for fitting this model are not necessarily straightforward (see Chapter 10 of Ramsay and Silverman 1997), although by using a grid of points in s, the coefficient functions can be closely approximated.

In the current release of the S+FDA library we integrate over the entire range of the independent variable. If, for example, we want to form predictions based upon all values of the independent variable prior to the current time, t, we would want to integrate over the range $(0, t)$. This is possible in S+FDA when both response and covariates are functional data, and finite element basis functions are used. See section Example with Functional Dependent and Independent Variables on page 115.

Classical least-squares models can also be fitted using specific values of the function argument. For example, one might predict final height by the height at ages 2 and 3.

Regularization

For simplicity, suppose we have only a single functional independent variable and consider the grid of points discussed above. Notice that as the number of grid points increases, then so does the prediction accuracy, until, when the number of grid points exceeds the number of observations, perfect prediction is obtained. While models with such a large number of grid points can be fitted, they are not interesting in the sense that the coefficient functions tend to be highly irregular and give little insight into how the predictor affects the mean. Moreover, while perfect prediction may be possible in the current sample, prediction for new subjects will generally be much less successful. Smoothing of the coefficients gives better insight into the effect of the predictors, because it can limit the degrees of freedom used in prediction, as well as helping to establish the true predictive capabilities of the linear model.

Smoothing in functional linear models can be obtained in the usual manner by adding a roughness penalty term. A typical roughness penalty term for a coefficient function $\beta(s)$ might be $\lambda \int (\beta''(s))^2 ds$,

where $\beta''(s)$ is the second derivative and λ is the penalty parameter, but roughness penalties based on any linear differential operator are possible. Notice that roughness penalties for coefficients for functional dependent variables are also possible and often desirable. See Chapters 9-11 of Ramsay and Silverman (1997) for details.

Functional Dependent and Independent Variables

More general models in which both the independent and the dependent variables are functions are also available. These take the form

$$y(t) = \beta_0(t) + \int (\beta_1(s, t)x_1(s) + \beta_2(s, t)x_2(s))ds + \varepsilon(t)$$

Here both the dependent and independent variables are functions, as are the coefficients and error terms. Notice, however, that all of the coefficient functions, save the intercept, are functions of two arguments. If it is assumed that these two argument functions are separable functions that can be written as the tensor products of two sets of basis functions, then we assume that these functions are of class fProdFunction. Otherwise, they are of class fFinElemFunction.

Relationship to Classical Linear Regression

Functional linear regression model reduce to classical linear regression models when both the independent and dependent variables are constant over the domain.

Models containing both functional and nonfunctional independent variables are also often of interest, regardless of whether the dependent variable is functional. In S+FDA, functions that are constant over their domain are always represented internally as functional variables with a basis of class "constantBasis". However, any numeric or factor variable can be used in a functional linear model in the same manner that it is used in the S-PLUS lm procedure.

It is useful to notice that if $x(s)$ is constant for all s (has a constantBasis basis), then $\beta(s, t)$ is constant with respect to s, and $\int \beta(s, t)x(s)ds$ is simply $\beta(t)x$, i.e., integration over s is not required. Similarly, if $y(t)$ is constant with respect to t, then t disappears in the coefficients for the independent variables and in the error term.

EXAMPLE WITH A FUNCTIONAL DEPENDENT VARIABLE

In this section we give an example of a functional linear model in which the dependent variable is the only functional variable. Our data is the height data first examined in Chapter 1. This is the data collected on the heights of 54 females and 39 males as they grew from age 1 to 18. In Chapter 1 the height data was used for a number of analyses, including a linear model predicting a patient's sex in terms of their growth function. Here we predict the patients growth as a function of their final height (to get an overall measure of growth), and their sex. As you may recall from Chapter 1, the functional variable fHgt gives the vector of growth curves for all individuals.

We begin by standardizing the growth curves so that all individuals grow by the same amount. We also create a data frame containing the height curves, the sex variable, and the final heights of all individuals. This is accomplished with the following statements:

```
> ratio <- 100/(heightData[31,2:94] - heightData[1,2:94])
> sHgt <- fHgt
> for(i in 1:93)
        sHgt[i] <- (fHgt[i]-heightData[1,i+1])*ratio[i]
> dataHgt <- data.frame(sHgt=sHgt,
                sex=as.factor(c(rep("F",54),rep("M",39))),
                finalHgt=t(heightData[31,2:94]))
```

The linear model can then be fitted using the function fLM as follows:

```
> predLm <- fLM(sHgt~-1+sex, dataHgt)
```

We next plot the fitted values for males and females using the fitted values returned by fLM:

```
> par(mfrow=c(2,1))
> plot(predLm$fitted[1], main="Fitted values")
> lines(predLm$fitted[55], lty=2)
> legend(1,100, c("females", "males"), lty=1:3)
> plot(fFunction(fFunction(predLm$fitted[1]),
        linDop=fDop(1)), main="Fitted values")
> lines(fFunction(fFunction(predLm$fitted[55]),
        linDop=fDop(1)), lty=2)
> legend(1,100, c("females", "males"), lty=1:3)
```

This result is displayed in Figure 6.1:

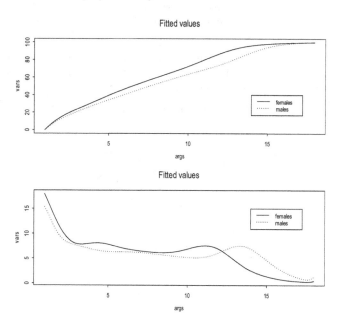

Figure 6.1: *Fitted female and male (standardized) growth curves (top) and derivatives (bottom).*

From the top graph in Figure 6.1, we see that if we standardize to a constant total growth for both males and females, then the males lag behind the females in their growth. The main reason for this is the longer period of male growth during adolescence of the males - since total growth has been standardized, the males growth continues after female growth stops, and thus must lag behind the females. Looking at the derivative curves in the bottom of the graph, we see that, as in Chapter 1, the rate of growth for the females shows a bump around age four that does not seem to be present in the males.

The object predLm created in the call to fLm above is an object of class "fLm". The model coefficients are returned as the coefficients component of predLm, where coefficients is a list objects of class "fProdFunction", each of which corresponds to a predictor (including the scalar predictors) in the model. Here there are two coefficient functions, the first is for the females, and the second is for the males. These coefficient functions can be plotted as follows:

```
> par(mfrow=c(1,1))
> plot(predLm$coef[[1]], main="coefficient Functions")
> lines(fMargin(predLm$coef[[2]],1), lty=2)
> legend(1,5.9, c("female", "male"), lty=1:2)
```

The resulting plot is given in Figure 6.2.

Coefficient Functions

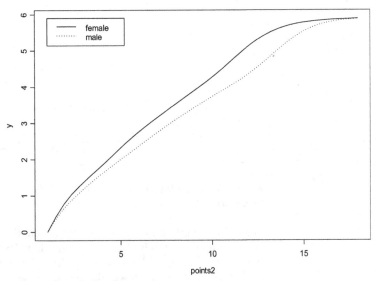

Figure 6.2: *Coefficient functions for the height data.*

As might be expected, the coefficient functions look somewhat like scaled versions of the fitted values shown in the top of Figure 6.1.

Modeling the Derivatives

Derivatives of functions can be used in a linear model in the same places that the function proper can be used. For example, the following fits and plots the first derivative of height, which give the same plot as bottom plot in Figure 6.1:

```
> DsHgt <- fVector(sHgt, linDop=fDop(1))
> dpredLm <- fLM(DsHgt ~ -1 + sex, dataHgt)
```

```
> plot(dpredLm$coef[[1]], xlab="age", ylab="hight",
        main="Derivative Coefficient Functions")
> lines(fMargin(dpredLm$coef[[2]],1), lty=2)
> legend(14,1, c("female", "male"), lty=1:2)
```

EXAMPLE WITH FUNCTIONAL INDEPENDENT VARIABLES

As an example with a functional independent variable, we consider the weather data. This is data collected on the (average) daily temperature and the daily precipitation of 35 Canadian weather stations over a one year period. Following Chapter 9 of Ramsay and Silverman (1997), we predict logarithm of the total yearly precipitation as a linear function of the daily temperature functions.

We first fit the model without a penalty function to see why a penalty is needed:

```
> predPrecip <- fLM(log(prec)~-1+fTemp, fWeather)
> plot(predPrecip$coef[[1]])
```

This resulting coefficient function for temperature is displayed in Figure 6.3.Coefficient functions for the height data

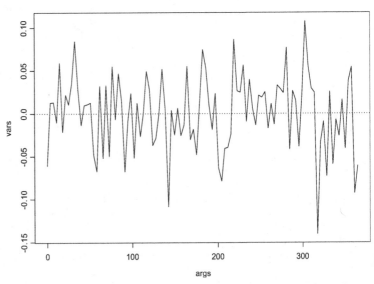

Figure 6.3: *Coefficient function for temperature when there is no penalty in the linear model.*

While the residual sum of squares vanishes, indicating perfect prediction, the coefficient function is highly irregular and nearly impossible to interpret - the model is badly overfitted.

Another measure of fit is the cross-validated prediction error. In cross-validation, the model is fitted with each observation, in turn, left out of the model. The predicted value for the deleted observation is then computed, and the *deleted residual* is computed by subtracting this predicted value from the observed value. The cross validation prediction error is then computed as the sum of the squared deleted residuals.

The cross-validated prediction error for this example can be computed as follows:

```
> crossValidLM <- function(xLambda, xPenMat, jMatx)
{
    fun <- function(i, fWeather, xLambda, xPenMat, jMatX)
    {
        ans <- fLM(log(prec)~-1+fTemp, fWeather[-i,],
                xPenalty=list(lambda=xLambda, linDop=fDop(2)),
                jMatX=jMatX, xPenMat=xPenMat)
        coefun <- fFunction(getCoef(ans$coef[[1]]),
                            ans$coef[[1]]$fBasis1)
        pred <- fInProd(fWeather$fTemp[i], coefun)
        log(fWeather$prec[i]) - pred
    }
    ans <- sapply(1:35, fun, fWeather=fWeather,
            xLambda=xLambda, xPenMat=xPenMat, jMatX=jMatX)
    sum(ans*ans)
}
> jMatX <- fInProd(getBasis(fWeather$fTemp),
                    getBasis(fWeather$fTemp))
> xPenMat <- fInProd(getBasis(fWeather$fTemp),
                    getBasis(fWeather$fTemp),
                    linDop1=fDop(2), linDop2=fDop(2))
```

In the crossValidLM function, the delete predicted values are computed by integrating the product of the lone independent variable and its coefficient function. The function requires two matrices, xPenMat and jMatX as input. These matrices depend only upon the basis of the functional independent variables, and thus do not change as observations are added or removed. The function fLM has been implemented so as to take advantage of these precomputed values in speeding up the computations.

To find an optimal penalty parameter, we executed the crossValidLM function over a grid of potential penalty parameters as follows:

```
> xLam <- c(0, 10^seq(1:10))
> bb <- double(11)
> for(i in 1:11)
        bb[i] <- crossValidLM(xLam[i], xPenMat, jMatx)
> plot(log(xLam+1), bb)
> lines(log(xLam+1), bb)
```

The resulting plot is shown in Figure 6.4.

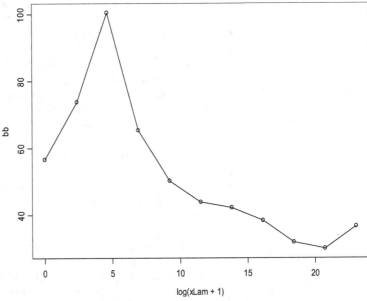

Figure 6.4: *Cross-validated sums of squares error for various values of the log of the penalty parameter (plus 1) on the horizontal axis.*

The value xLam = 0 corresponds to no smoothing, and the corresponding cross-validated prediction error is 56.61. Smoothing the coefficients during the estimation procedure yields more accurate results. The smallest cross validation prediction error was 32.02 corresponding to xLam = 10^9 :

```
> predPrecipPen <- fLM(log(prec)~-1+fTemp, fWeather,
              xPenalty=list(lambda=10^9, linDop=fDop(2)),
              jMatX=jMatX, xPenMat=xPenMat)
> plot(predPrecipPen$coef[[1]])
```

A plot of the fitted coefficient function for this value of xLam is given in Figure 6.5. From this figure we see that the coefficient function gives moderately negative weights to temperatures around May, and highly positive weights to temperatures around September, with a small positive weights to temperatures around January.

A plot of the predicted versus the actual values is obtained as follows:

```
> plot(getCoef(predPrecipPen$fitted), log(fWeather$prec),
        xlab="Predicted Values", ylab="Observed Values")
> lines(rbind(c(5,5), c(7.5,7.5)))
```

Here we use the function getCoef to extract the scalar fitted values from the fitted value functions of class "constantBasis". The plot is shown in Figure 6.6. Although there is an apparent outlier, removing it has little effect on the fitted model.

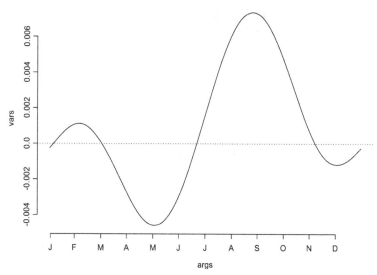

Figure 6.5: *The fitted coefficients function for temperature with penalty parameter10^9.*

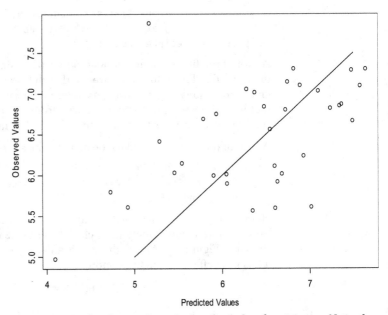

Figure 6.6: *Predicted versus observed values for the log of precipitation. Notice the outlier near (5, 7.5).*

EXAMPLE WITH FUNCTIONAL DEPENDENT AND INDEPENDENT VARIABLES

It is also possible to fit functional linear models in which both the dependent and independent variables are functional. This section gives two examples that differ in the domain of integration for the independent variable:

- over the whole interval $[0, T]$

- the *historical* model, in which the independent variable is integrated over the range $[s_0(t), t]$, where $s_0(t)$ is a lag before time t.

gaitarray **Data Set**

The following example is taken from Chapter 12 of Ramsay and Silverman (1997). The data set was originally collected at the Motion Analysis Laboratory at Children's Hospital in San Diego (see Olshen, et al., 1989), and consists of measurements of the angles made by the hip and by the knee of each of 39 children. The angles are measured over 20 time points through the course of one gait cycle. Time has been normalized over the gait cycle for each child. The three dimensional 20 by 39 by 2 array, gaitarray, contains both of these matrices, with the first matrix in the array being hip angle.

Here we use a Fourier basis with nineteen basis functions to obtain an object of data frame fGait.

```
> fGaitBasis <- fBasis(type="Fourier", fDomain=c(0,1),
                         nbasis=19)
> gaitNames <- list(NormalizedTime=gaittime,
                      Cases=seq(dim(gaitarray)[2]),
                        Angle="deg")
> fHipVec <- fVector(object=fGaitBasis, y=fHip,
                      fArgs=gaittime, fNames=gaitNames)
> fKneeVec <- fVector(object=fGaitBasis, y=fKnee,
                       fArgs=gaittime, fNames=gaitNames)
> fGait <- data.frame(fHip=fHipVec,fKnee=fKneeVec)
```

Since there are only twenty sampling points, a nineteen basis functions fit the children's curves very well - the maximum difference between the fitted curve and the observed measurement is 0.00082. Because we have standardized with respect to time, the domain of the functions (argument fDomain) is the interval (0,1).

In our example, we predict knee angle (fGait$fKnee) in terms of hip angle (fGait$fHip).

No smoothing

We begin our analysis by computing the solution without explicit smoothing. The code for fitting the model:

```
> predKnee <- fLM(fGait$fKnee ~ fGait$fHip)
```

By default, an intercept is included in the model. The fitted model contains two coefficient functions, a function for the intercept, and a functional data object of class "fProdFunction" for knee angle. These functions are obtained as the first and second elements, respectively, of the list of coefficients predKneeU$coefficients. We plot the data, the coefficients for knee angle, the fitted values, and the residuals:

```
> par(mfrow=c(2,2))
> plot(fGait$fKnee, main="Response Functions")
> plot(predKnee$coef[[2]])
> title(main="Bivariate Coefficient Function")
> plot(predKnee$fitted, main="Predicted Functions")
> plot(predKnee$resid, main="Residual Functions")
```

The resulting plot is given in Figure 6.7. It is evident that the coefficient function for hip angle, the bivariate function in the upper right corner, is quite irregular.

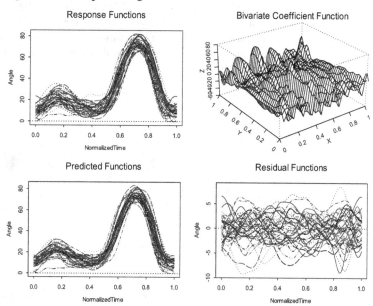

Figure 6.7: *Top left: knee angle functions (response). Clockwise from top right: hip angle coefficients, fitted values, and residuals from an unsmoothed fit.*

Smoothing

While the unsmoothed results are useful for prediction, the highly irregular shape of the coefficient matrix gives little insight into how the hip and knee angles are related. Moreover, the cross-validated prediction error may be less than optimal. Function fLM provides for two smoothing parameters, one for the independent variables and another for the dependent variables. Some experimentation with these parameters yielded much smoother coefficient estimates, while at the same time having little effect on the magnitude of the residuals.

```
> predKneeSmoothed <- fLM(fGait$fKnee ~ fGait$fHip,
            xPenalty=list(lambda=0.1, linDop=fDop(2)),
            yPenalty=list(lambda=0.000001, linDop=fDop(2)))
```

This result is displayed in Figure 6.8. From the figure, we see that the bivariate coefficient function predicting knee angle as a function of hip angle are much smoother.

Conceptually, the two smoothing parameters could be handled by cross validation, but the computational cost increases dramatically with the number of parameters to be estimated. When the dependent variable is scalar, it is possible to do cross validation on the scalar residuals, as illustrated above. And for functional dependent variables, the residuals are functions with values in the same domain as the dependent variable, so that there is a choice of cross validation smoothing criteria.

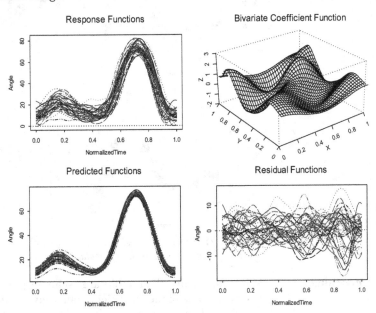

Figure 6.8: *Top left: knee angle functions (response). Clockwise from top right: hip angle coefficients, fitted values, and residuals from a smoothed fit.*

lip **Data Set**   The following example is taken from Chapter 10 of Ramsay and Silverman (1997). The data set was originally collected at the Haskins Speech Laboratories at Yale University by V. Gracco. The considerable preprocessing is described in Ramsay and Silverman, and in Malfait and Ramsay. The S-PLUS data set lip consists of four variables: EMG, acceleration, position, time.

The goal here is to model lip acceleration, acceleration, as a function of EMG activity EMG. To fit the historic linear model, we first create an object fLip with 101 Fourier basis functions in the time domain $[0, 690]$

```
> fLipBasis <- fBasis(type="Fourier", fDomain=c(0, 690),
                      nbasis=101)
> fLip <- list(time=lip$time, fEmg=fVector(fLipBasis,
                  lip$emg, lip$time), fAcc=fVector(fLipBasis,
                  lip$acc, lip$time))
```

No Smoothing   The code to fit the historic linear model without explicit smoothing:

```
> lip.hlm <- fLMFinElem(fAcc~fEmg, data=fLip, param=11,
                       lag=4)
```

in which param is a parameter to specify the number of elements in the domain of each argument of the bivariate regression function. With param = 11, lag can be an integer range from 1 and 11. lag is a parameter to specify $\delta = lag \cdot \Delta_x$ in the lower bound of

$$s_0(t) = max(0, t - \delta),$$ where Δ_x is the lag length of each triangle element used in basis functions. By default, an intercept is included in the model. The fitted model lip.hlm contains a list, named fBeta, of the functional data objects with class fFinElemFunction. The fitted values and residuals can be estimated by the predict method:

```
> predfLip <- predict(lip.hlm, fLip$time)
```

We plot the data and the estimated bivariate regression function:

```
> par(mfrow=c(2,2))
> plot(fLip$fAcc)
> title("Functional Data fAcc")
> plot(lip.hlm$fBeta)
> title("Estimated Regression Function")
```

The fitted values and the residuals can be plotted by making choices 1 (for predicted value) and 2 (for residuals) in the menu produced by the command:

```
> plot(predfLip)
```

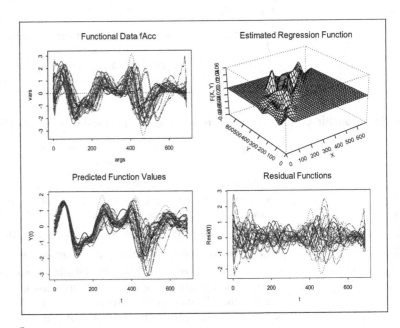

Figure 6.9: *Top left: lip acceleration (response), Clockwise from top right: estimated regression function with lag=4, fitted values, and residuals from an unsmoothed fit.*

Smoothing

To smooth the shape of the regression function, fLMFinElem provides a smoothing parameter lambda. This produces smoother coefficient estimates, while at the same time having little effect on the magnitude of the residuals.

```
> lip.hlms <- fLMFinElem(fAcc~fEmg, data=fLip, param=11,
                         lambda=50000, lag=4)
> predliphlms <- predict(lip.hlms, fLip$time)
```

The results are displayed in. Note the smoother regression function, compared withFigure 6.9:

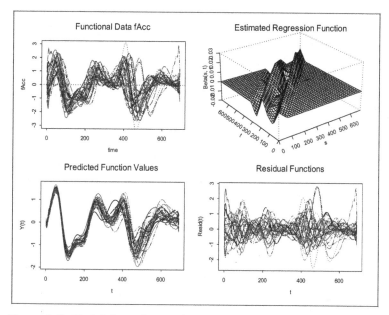

Figure 6.10: *Top left: lip acceleration (response), Clockwise from top right: estimated regression function with lag=4, fitted values, and residuals from an unsmoothed fit.*

FUNCTIONAL GENERALIZED LINEAR MODELS

7

In functional linear models, the residuals are assumed to be independent Gaussian random variables with a constant variance. However, in many cases independence is adequate to insure unbiased estimates. If the dependent variable is from some other probability distribution (e.g. binomial, Poisson, or gamma), then a generalized linear model is appropriate. S+FDA provides a function fGLM to fit functional generalized linear models in which the dependent variable is a scalar. It is not currently possible in S+FDA to fit functional generalized linear models in which the dependent variable is a function.

WEATHER EXAMPLE

The example involves daily average temperature and precipitation measurements taken at 35 Canadian weather stations over the course of a year. Functional data was obtained from this weather data using a Fourier basis with 101 basis functions. Although some smoothing occurred when the functional data was created since fewer basis functions were used than the number of observation points (365), additional smoothing was required.

We divided the 35 weather stations into two groups, representing coastal and interior cities, respectively.

Modeling the Grouped Data

We fit a functional logistic classification model to one of the groups of stations to predict group membership. The fit for the coastal region is accomplish as follows. We first define the coastal weather station indicator variables, yCoastal, and then fit a functional generalized linear model predicting this Bernoulli indicator in terms of both the average daily temperature and precipitation functions at the respective weather stations:

```
> Cities <- row.names(fWeather)
> CoastalCities <- c("Charlottetown", "Churchill",
        "Halifax", "Iqaluit", "Prince Rupert", "Resolute",
        "Saint Johns",  "Sydney", "Vancouver",
        "Victoria", "Yarmouth")
> yCoastal <-as.numeric(as.logical(match(Cities,
                        CoastalCities,nomatch=0)))
> glmCoastal <- fGLM(yCoastal ~ fTemp + fPrec,
                family=binomial, data=fWeather,
                penalty=list(lambda=10000, linDop=fDop(2)))
```

We use a single smoothing parameter, lambda, selected with a minimum of experimentation. Although two penalty parameters would be desirable because there are two predictors, this is not yet possible in the S+FDA module. cross validation could be used to select the penalty parameters, but this is more expensive than in the functional linear model case because functional generalized linear models require iterative algorithms.

Interpreting the Results

Figure 7.1 shows that the fitted values for the models are all close to 0 or 1 and perfectly predict their groups.

```
> par(mfrow=c(1, 1))
> plot(glmCoastal$fitted, type="n", ylim=c(-.1, 1.1),
       xlab="observation number", ylab="")
#true classes
> points(yCoastal, pch=1, cex=1.5)
#fitted values
> points(glmCoastal$fitted, pch=18, cex=1)
> abline(h=c(0, 1))
> title("Fitted Values")
```

Fitted Values

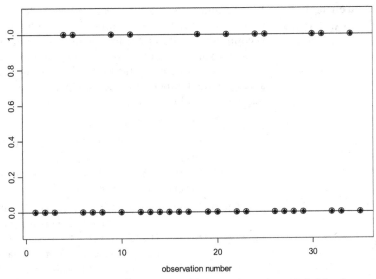

Figure 7.1: *Fitted values (diamonds) and binary response (open circles) for the logistic model of weather data for coastal vs. interior cities.*

However, since there are only 35 weather stations and 365 functional predictors (one independent variables for each day of the year), the fit of the values used to define the models is an overly optimistic estimate of their predictive ability. Below we evaluate the models using cross validation.

Cross Validation

While it requires significant computation time, cross validation (also known in this context as the leaving-out-one method - see Lackenbruch, 1977) can be used to evaluate the classification produced from the generalized linear model. Here we use cross-validation to obtain a misclassification matrix:

```
> crossValidGLM <- function(lambda, y)
{
    fun <- function(i, fWeather, lambda)
    {
        ans <- fGLM(y ~ fTemp + fPrec, family=binomial,
                    data=fWeather[-i, ],
                    penalty=list(lambda=lambda,
                                 linDop=fDop(2)))
        cat(i, " ")
        getCoef(ans$coef[[1]]) * 365 +
                fInProd(ans$coef[[2]], fWeather$fTemp[i],
                        eps=0.00001) +
                fInProd(ans$coef[[3]], fWeather$fPrec[i],
                        eps=0.00001)
    }
    dd <- data.frame(y=y, fTemp=fWeather$fTemp,
                     fPrec=fWeather$fPrec)
    sapply(1:35, fun, fWeather=dd, lambda=lambda)
}
```

The predicted value is computed as the sum of three terms (one for each coefficient): a constant term (times the length of the domain of the functions, the integral of a constant) and two integrals, one for the average daily temperature functions times the temperature coefficient function, and one for the precipitation times the precipitation coefficient function.

Predicted values for the coastal region logistic model can be computed as follows:

```
> predCoastal <- crossValidGLM(10000, y=yCoastal)
> muCoastal <- binomial()$inverse(predCoastal)
```

We then use the predicted values (muCoastal) to compute the probabilities of correct classification for the models defined by each of the four groups, taking an observation to be classified in that group if its predicted value is greater than 0.5. The results are plotted as follows and displayed in Figure 7.2:

```
> par(mfrow=c(1,1))
> plot(glmCoastal$fitted, type="n", ylim=c(-.1, 1.1),
        xlab="observation number", ylab="")
#true classes
> points(yCoastal, pch=1, cex=1.5)
# cross-validated estimates
> points(muCoastal, pch=4, cex=1)
> abline(h=c(0,1))
> title("Cross-validated Predictions")
```

Crossvalidated Predictions

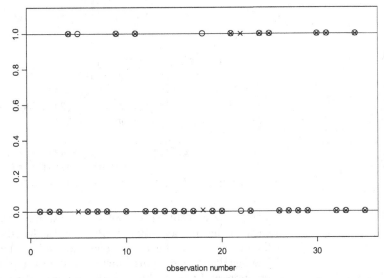

Figure 7.2: *Cross-validated predictions (crosses) and binary response (open circles).*

Only 3 (Churchill, Prince Rupert, Schefferville) out of 35 weather stations are misclassified, giving a cross-validated error rate of less that 1%:

```
> Cities[(muCoastal > 0.5 & !yCoastal) |
          (muCoastal < 0.5 & yCoastal)]
```

POLYCHOTOMOUS CLASSIFICATION

Polychotomous classification models are not currently available for classification in S+FDA. When there are more than two groups, the strategy of fitting a logistic model to each group and classifying according to best prediction may work. Note that with this method an observation could be classified into more than one group, or even fail to be classified into any group.

FUNCTIONAL PRINCIPAL COMPONENTS

8

Classical principal components analysis is used in many ways, including analyzing data complexity, reducing data dimension, studying relationships between variables, clustering observations, and interpreting variances and covariances in multivariate analysis. These same uses are also important in functional principal components analysis, but in functional principal components the number of "variables" in the analysis is infinite, so that reduction to a finite number of principal component scores is the only way to make the computation tractable. Functional principal component loadings are also functions, and it may be desirable or even necessary to regularize or smooth them. Historically, principal components extracted from functional data are called *harmonics*.

The basic idea in functional principal components analysis is to find functions whose inner products with the data yield the maximum variation in the curves. The first principal component accounts for the most variation, the second principal component accounts for the largest variation orthogonal to the first principal component, and so on. In this way, much of the variation in the random data can be captured using only a few principal components.

Specifically, in classical multivariate analysis, if x is a random variable, the first principal component is the unit vector α_1 that maximizes the variance of the linear combination or inner product $\alpha_1^T x$. In general the i th principal component is the unit vector that maximizes the variance of the inner product $\alpha_i^T x$, and is orthogonal to all of the previous principal components. There are a maximum of p principal components, where p is the dimension of x.

In functional data, the inner product is defined by integration. For a single random function $x(t)$, the process of determining functional principal components is equivalent to selecting a grid of points in t, say $t_1, t_2, ..., t_m$, where $t_1 < t_2 < ... < t_m$, computing the classical principal components of the vector $x = (x(t_1), x(t_2), ..., x(t_m))^T$, and then letting the grid size decrease to zero (and yielding an infinite number of variables). Notice that, in theory, any number of principal components can be computed, although in practice the number of important principal components (those with "large" variances) will be small.

Specified as integrals, for a random functions $x(t)$, the ith principal component is the function $\alpha_i(t)$ that maximizes the variance of the principal component score $Z_i = \int \alpha_i(t)x(t)dt$ and satisfies the constraints $\int \alpha_i(t)\alpha_i(t)dt = 1$ and $\int \alpha_i(t)\alpha_j(t) = 0$ for $j < i$. For two functional variables $x(t)$ and $y(t)$, the ith principal component maximizes the variance of the random variable

$Z_i = \int \alpha_{ix}(t)x(t)dt + \int \alpha_{iy(t)}x(t)dt$ subject to the normality constraint

$\int \alpha_{ix}(t)\alpha_{ix}(t)dt + \int \alpha_{iy}(t)\alpha_{iy}(t)dt = 1$, and to orthogonality

constraints $\int \alpha_{ix}(t)\alpha_{jx}(t)dt + \int \alpha_{iy}(t)\alpha_{jy}(t)dt = 0$ for all $j < i$.
Principal components with three or more functional varieties are handled by extension.

As in the classical case, functional principal components are computed by obtaining a sample of realizations of the random function, say $x_j(t), j = 1, ..., n$, and then computing estimates of the functions $\alpha_i(t)$ based upon the variances and covariances observed in this sample.

Centering

Centering, or subtraction of the mean, is usually performed prior to extracting harmonics (principal components) because the interest is usually in maximizing variances about the mean function. It is also possible and common for researchers to compute "principal components" from the uncentered data. However, if the mean function is not everywhere zero, the largest principal component obtained from this uncentered data is usually closely related to the mean function. Although the extracted "principal components" no longer reflect the linear combination with maximum variance (they are not really principal components), they may still prove useful.

Standardization

Analogous to classical multivariate analysis, it may sometimes be desirable to standardize the functions by centering and transforming the sample variance of each function (at each point in its domain) to a variance of 1. This is akin to computing principal components on the correlation matrix rather than on the variance-covariance matrix. Notice, however, that standardization is not always possible. For example, in some problems the random functions have restricted endpoints and thus have a variance of zero at their endpoints with the variance decreasing to zero in a regular manner as the endpoints are approached (see Figure 8.1). As a consequence the standardized functions are not defined at their endpoints, and may exhibit undesirable behavior in nearby regions. In order to standardize, the principal components would have to be computed over a reduced domain. This option is not available in the current implementation of S+FDA.

In the following we give an example based upon bone shapes. We begin by describing how the data was collected and how the functions we will use were derived from the given data. We then give a brief technical discussion of functional principal components. Finally, we give a complete principal-component analysis of the functional data.

ANALYSIS OF THE BONE SHAPE DATA

Our example is from archeology, although the techniques could also be used to study medical aspects of modern humans. The analysis is similar to that given in Chapter 6 of Ramsay and Silverman (2002). The data was collected on 96 femur bones from 60 individuals originally buried at St. Peter's Church in the north of England. Some individuals had both their left and right femurs analyzed. The data is concerned with the two dimensional shape of the *interchondylar* notch, located in the femur at the knee. It was collected using a two-dimensional x-ray of the notch, and consists a bone identifier, two vectors containing the x and y coordinates of the bone notch outline (from the x-ray), an indicator for male (TRUE is male), older (TRUE is older), and eb, an indicator of eburnation (TRUE indicates the presence of a polished bone surface caused by the complete loss of cartilage).

The x and y coordinates are measured in pixels, and were collected as follows: For each x location the two value(s) of y corresponding to the notch outline are noted.

Graphs of the first ten notch curves are given in Figure 8.1. The S-PLUS code used to produce these plots is as follows:

```
> apply(boneNotch[, c("x","y")], 2, range)
       x   y
[1,]  19  66
[2,] 102 125
> par(mfrow=c(1, 1))
> plot(19, 66, type="n", xlim=c(19,102), ylim=c(66,125),
       xlab="x", ylab="y")

> boneTmp <- split(boneNotch,boneNotch$boneID)
> dummy <- lapply(boneTmp[1:10], function(z) {
               imin <- min((1:length(z$y))[z$y==min(z$y)])
               yy <- z$y
               yy[1:imin] <- -yy[1:imin]
               ii <- order(yy)
               lines(z$x[ii], z$y[ii], type="l")
             })
```

Notice that in these curves, the femur bone is below the curve, and that only the interchondylar notch is displayed in Figure 8.1.

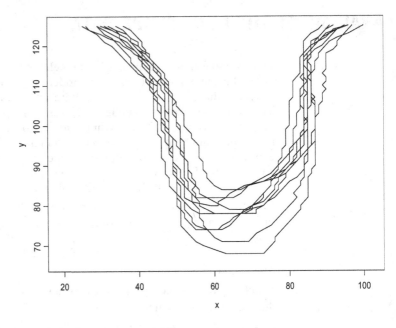

Figure 8.1: *The first ten bone notch curves.*

Registration

Registration is the process of eliminating uninteresting differences between the curves. The need for registration is apparent from Figure 8.1: each bone notch starts and ends at a different x location, and the depth of each bone notch is different. Because starting and ending x locations, notch depth, and curve orientation (due to whether the left or right leg is measured) are partially artifacts of the way that the data is gathered (the location of the bone on the x-ray), these differences need to be eliminated prior to performing the analysis of interest. Differences between curves based upon measuring the left or right leg have already been eliminated by reflecting the curve through the vertical axis. For these curves, the data extraction process (discussed below) eliminates the remaining differences. It should be noted that curve registration must be carried out with caution, because curve differences that were not present in the original data could be introduced in the process.

Extracting the Functions

The S-PLUS code used to extract the data is given in the help file for `boneData` and is not reproduced here. Interested users should consult this help file for details of the extraction.

Because it is not possible to represent each bone notch curve as a single function (there may be two y values for each x value), here we use two functions $x(t)$ and $y(t)$ giving the x and y coordinates of the curve as a function of the distance along the curve (t) starting at the left-most endpoint. The process of extracting these functions begins by standardizing the x and y values by subtracting the minimum and dividing by the range. All of the resulting curves start at $(0,1)$, end at $(1,0)$, and reach a minimum along the x axis. The x and y coordinates are then sorted.

Rather than using the raw data values, adjacent values are averaged to provide a modest amount of smoothing. The distance along the curve is computed as the cumulative sum of the distances between each of the points on the averaged curve. These distances are then standardized so that each curve begins at $t = 0$ and ends at $t = 1$. The functional data objects $x(t)$ and $y(t)$ are computed from the standardized distances using the `fFunction` constructor.

We use a B-spline basis of order 4 with ten basis functions is to represent the $x(t)$ and $y(t)$ components of each bone notch curve. Because there are only 10 basis functions, projection onto the basis results into additional smoothing.

The functions $x(t)$ and $y(t)$ are placed into objects of class "fVector", called `boneVecX` and `boneVecY`, respectively, each having 96 functions, one function for each bone notch. We then create the `boneData` data frame from these "fVector" objects and the `older`, `male`, and `eb` predictors found in the raw bone data. The `boneData` data frame is included with the S+FDA library. Additional details on the conversion of the raw data into its functional form are given in Chapter 6 of Ramsay and Silverman (2002).

The `fPlotCycle` command is used to plot the x functions against the y functions for the same argument values:

```
> fPlotCycle(boneData$boneVecX[1:10],
             boneData$boneVecY[1:10])
```

The resulting plot is displayed in Figure 8.2.

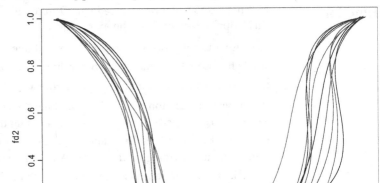

Figure 8.2: *The first ten smoothed and registered bone notch curves.*

Although these curves have been registered as discussed above, additional registration may be desirable, because each curve may cover slightly different portions of the notch, and the orientation of each notch may vary from one curve to the next (the x-ray used to obtain the curve may have a slightly different orientation). We ignore these considerations in our analysis.

Principal Components

In the following command the function fPCA is used to extract the first ten harmonics (principal components) from the bone notch curves in the boneData data frame:

```
> bonePCA <- fPCA(~boneVecX+boneVecY, boneData, nharm=10,
                  center=T)
```

Here we simultaneously extract principal components for both functional vectors boneVecX and boneVecY. Recall that these functions give the x and y locations of the curves as a function of the distance along the curve from the left end point, the curve length.

Interpretation   The bonePCA object created above is an object of class "fPCA". The eigenvalues corresponding to each of the extracted harmonics are returned as the vector values. These give the variance of the corresponding harmonic. The proportion of the total variance explained by the harmonic is returned as the vector varprop. The order is such that the proportion of variance explained by the first harmonic is largest. The cumulative proportions of the variances are computed using the command:

```
> round(cumsum(bonePCA$varprop), 3)
```

which results in the following output:

```
  PC1   PC2   PC3   PC4   PC5   PC6   PC7   PC8
0.456 0.751 0.869 0.912 0.948 0.974 0.984 0.989
  PC9 PC10
0.993 0.996
```

The first three harmonics are clearly the most important, accounting for 86.9 percent of the total variation in the 96 pairs of functions. These three harmonics can be plotted using the command plot(bonePCA). However, because we simultaneously extracted the harmonics from the two functions $x(t)$ and $y(t)$, for this data, it is easiest to interpret the harmonics if they are plotted about the mean of the bone notch curves, which can be accomplished as follows. We first standardize the harmonic to the amount of variance it explains by multiplying the harmonic coefficients by the square root of the corresponding eigenvalues:

```
> harmCoef <- getCoef(bonePCA$harmonics[1:3]) %*%
                      diag(sqrt(bonePCA$values[1:3]))
> harm <- fVector(harmCoef,getBasis(bonePCA$harmonics),
                  getNames(bonePCA$harmonics))
```

The mean functions for boneVecX and boneVecY (from which the harmonics were extracted) are then extracted from the bonePCA object using the getComponent function for obtaining the components of a composite basis:

```
> meanX <- getComponent(bonePCA$fMean, 1)
> meanY <- getComponent(bonePCA$fMean, 2)
```

A composite basis is currently created for the means and the harmonics for computational reasons. In the future these components will be split out, and a list of functional components will be returned.

Plotting the Harmonic Loadings

We are now in a position to plot the first three harmonics. Usually the `plot.fPCA` function would be used, but here we have two related functions, and so a cycle plot is preferred. Plotting is accomplished as follows:

```
> par(mfrow=c(3, 1))
> percnt <- c(45.6, 29.5, 11.8)
> for (i in 1:3) {
        x1 <- fFunction(getComponent(harm[i], 1))
        x <- fVector(meanX, meanX + x1, meanX - x1)
        y1 <- fFunction(getComponent(harm[i], 2))
        y <- fVector(meanY, meanY + y1, meanY - y1)
        fPlotCycle(x,y)
        title(paste("Bone Data P.C.", i, "\n", percnt[i],
                "% of the Variance"))
}
```

The "fVector" objects x and y contain the function mean, and the mean plus or minus the harmonic coefficients, for each harmonic. The command `fPlotCycle(x,y)` plots the vector of functions, as shown in Figure 8.3:

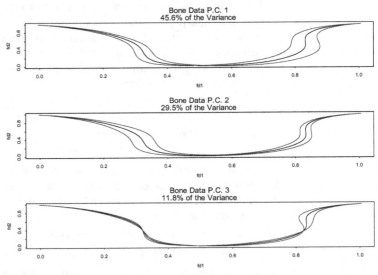

Figure 8.3: *Variation of the first three harmonics about the function mean.*

The offset (in the x or y direction) from the mean gives the magnitude of the principal component loading at each point in the curve. Values above or to the right of the mean indicate a positive impact on the principal component score, while values below or to the left of the mean indicate a negative impact.

Close inspection of Figure 8.3, reveals that the offset is positive prior to the minimum, and negative after the minimum, with the highest magnitudes along the sides of the notch. Thus the first harmonic seems to measure a left or right shift in the notch. This is a possible indication that the data needs further registration.

The second harmonic looks very much like the first harmonic, but all of the loadings are positive, concentrated on the notch walls, with more emphasis on the left notch wall. This seems to be a measure of the notch width.

The third harmonic has near zero loadings everywhere, except near the top of the right notch wall. Some curves are indented near this location. This harmonic seems to be a measure of this indentation in the right notch wall.

Plotting the Mean Curves

Another plot that is useful in understanding the principal components is to plot the mean curves for a specified range of harmonic scores on each harmonic. Here we plot the overall mean curve, the mean of the curves with scores in the quantile range (0.60, 0.90) (on the first harmonic), and the mean of the curves with scores in the quantile range (0.10, 0.40):

```
> par(mfrow=c(3, 1))
> for(i in 1:3) {
      q <- quantile(bonePCA$scores[, 1],
                  probs=c(0.9, 0.6, 0.4, 0.1))
      y <- bonePCA$scores[,i]
      iu <- y < q[1] & y > q[2]
      il <- y < q[3] & y > q[4]
      ansX <- fVector(meanX,mean(boneData$boneVecX[il]),
                            mean(boneData$boneVecX[iu]))
      ansY <- fVector(meanY,mean(boneData$boneVecY[il]),
                            mean(boneData$boneVecY[iu]))
      fPlotCycle(ansX, ansY)
      title(paste("Bone Data P.C. ", i, "\nMeans Curves"))
  }
```

The resulting plots are given in Figure 8.4.

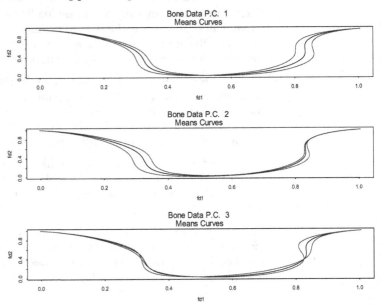

Figure 8.4: *The mean bone curves for harmonic scores in a specified range.*

The curves look much like the harmonic curves in Figure 8.3.

Specifying a Rotation

As in classical multivariate data analysis, the harmonics are not unique - they can be rotated. The resulting *rotated* harmonics no longer maximize the variance (though the total variance they explain remains unchanged), but they are potentially simpler to interpret because the rotation criteria that is used is chosen such that the resulting loadings exhibit *simple* structure - they tend to be either large in magnitude, or they are close to zero. The simplest rotation can be accomplished as follows:

```
> rotateBonePCA <- rotate(bonePCA, nharm=3)
```

Once the functional principal components have been rotated, a plot of the coefficients can be obtained using a simple modification of the code above:

```
# Standardize the harmonic coefficients
> rharm <- rotateBonePCA$harmonics
```

```
> rharmCoef <- getCoef(rharm)
> rharmCoef <- rharmCoef%*%diag(sqrt(bonePCA$values[1:3]))
> rharm <-fVector(rharmCoef, getBasis(rharm),
                  getNames(rharm))

# Plot the rotated harmonics
> par(mfrow=c(3, 1))
> percnt <- c(31.7, 31.1, 11.8)
> for (i in 1:3) {
      x1 <- fFunction(getComponent(rharm[i], 1))
      x <- fVector(meanX, meanX+x1, meanX-x1)
      y1 <- fFunction(getComponent(rharm[i], 2))
      y <- fVector(meanY, meanY+y1, meanY-y1)
      fPlotCycle(x,y)
      title(paste("Bone Data P.C.", i, "\n", percnt[i],
            "% of the Variance"))
  }
```

The resulting plot is displayed in Figure 8.5.

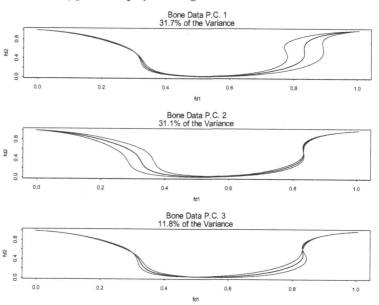

Figure 8.5: *The rotated principal functions.*

143

For the rotated loadings, the first harmonic measures the indentation in the right notch wall, the second harmonic measures the indentation in the left notch wall, and the third harmonic measures asymmetry in the notch. Notice that the roles of the first and third harmonic are switched from the unrotated case and that the indentation in the right notch wall now exhibits a much larger magnitude, while the asymmetry measure (the third rotated harmonic) is now much smaller in magnitude.

CANONICAL CORRELATION

9

Classical canonical correlation analysis finds linear transformations of two sets of variables that maximize the correlation between the transformed variables. If $x(t)$ and $y(t)$ are two functions defined on the same interval domain, functional canonical correlation analysis seeks coefficient or weight functions $w_x(t)$ and $w_y(t)$ that maximize the correlations between the random canonical variables

$W = \int w_x(t)x(t)dt$ and $Z = \int w_y(t)y(t)dt$. Functional canonical correlation analysis provides a mechanism for investigating the relationship of the variability of the two functions.

In the classical case, the canonical correlations are computed by solving a generalized eigenvalue problem, and a similar method is used for functional canonical correlations. And as in the classical case, additional canonical coefficients can be determined, orthogonal (uncorrelated) to those already found.

ANALYSIS OF THE GAIT DATA

Here we consider gait data described in the chapter on functional linear models (and in Chapter 12 of Ramsay and Silverman 1997) consisting of measurements of the angles made by the hip and by the knee of each of 39 children at twenty time points in a single stride or gait cycle.

The gait basis is a an object of class "FourierBasis" on the domain (0,1) with 21 basis functions:

```
> fGaitBasis <- fBasis(type="Fourier", fDomain=c(0,1),
                        nbasis=19)
> gaitNames <- list(NormalizedTime=gaittime,
                    Cases=seq(dim(gaitarray)[2]), Angle="deg")

> fHipVec <- fVector(object=fGaitBasis,y=fHip,
                        fArgs=gaittime, fNames=gaitNames)
> fKneeVec <- fVector(object=fGaitBasis,y=fKnee,
                        fArgs=gaittime, fNames=gaitNames)

> fGait <- data.frame(hip=fHipVec, knee=fKneeVec)
```

Since there are only 20 measurements over the gait cycle, the basis adequately captures all of the information collected with no error.

Because we have standardized with respect to time, the domain of the functions (argument fDomain) is the interval (0,1). The resulting functions can be plotted as follows:

```
> par(mfrow=c(2,1))
> plot(fGait[,"hip"], main="Hip Angle")
> plot(fGait[,"knee"], main="Knee Angle")
```

The display is shown in Figure 9.1

Next, we compute and plot the coefficient functions $w_x(t)$ and $w_y(t)$ for the canonical correlations using S+FDA statements:

```
> gaitCancor <- fCancor(fGait[,1], fGait[,2])
> plot(gaitCancor, main="No Smoothing")
```

The result is displayed in Figure 9.2. Note that the coefficient or weight functions are highly variable.

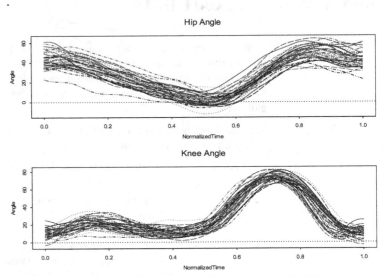

Figure 9.1: *Plot of the hip (top) and knee (bottom) angles for 39 children as they walk.*

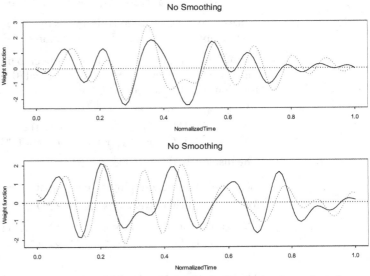

Figure 9.2: *Canonical function coefficient for the first (top) and second set of canonical coefficient functions. The solid curve corresponds to the hip data.*

In this unsmoothed analysis, all of the canonical correlations are close to 1. The reason for this can be seen by considering conventional methods. In a conventional canonical correlation analysis, we would evaluate each of the 39 knee and hip angle functions over a vector of time points $t_i, i = 1, ..., p$, and would then compute the canonical correlations over the p sets of variates for the hip and knee angles. A necessary condition for the p-dimensional variance-covariance matrix between the hip and knee variables to be nonsingular is that the number of observations be greater than $2p + 1$, otherwise there would in most cases be an infinite number of linear transformations for which canonical correlation would be equal to 1.

In a functional canonical correlation analysis, the grid of points becomes arbitrarily large, so that usually a infinite number of weight functions would result in a functional canonical correlation equal to 1.

Regularization To avoid such overfitting in the canonical correlation analysis, we *regularize* or smooth the canonical coefficients by applying a penalty function. One possibility for choosing the penalty parameter is to use cross validation, and define the score for a given penalty parameter to be the correlation of the canonical correlations obtained by deleting each observation is turn. The penalty parameter is then chosen so as to maximize this correlation (see Section 12.2.3 of Ramsay and Silverman, 1997).

The following computes the cross-validated correlations for six values of the penalty parameter (denoted by the lambda component of the xPenalty argument). Some preliminary exploration was involved in choosing to these six values appropriately.

```
> crossValid <- function(lambda)
{
  fun <- function(i, fGait, lambda)
  {
      pen <- list(lambda=lambda, linDop=fDop(2))
      ans <- fCancor(fGait[-i, 1],fGait[-i, 2],
                      xPenalty=pen, yPenalty=pen, ncan=1)
      c(fInProd(ans$xWeight[1], fGait[i, 1]),
        fInProd(ans$yWeight[1], fGait[i, 2]))
  }
  ans <- sapply(1:39, fun, fGait=fGait, lambda=lambda)
```

```
    cor(t(ans))[1,2]
    }
> xLam <- seq(from=5.e-6, to=5.e-5, by=5.e-6)
> aa <- double(length(xLam))
> for(i in 1:length(xLam))
        aa[i] <- crossValid(xLam[i])

> par(mfrow=c(1, 1))
> plot(xLam, aa, type="l")
> points(xLam, aa)
```

The resulting plot of the cross-validated correlations versus the penalty parameter value lambda is shown in Figure 9.3.

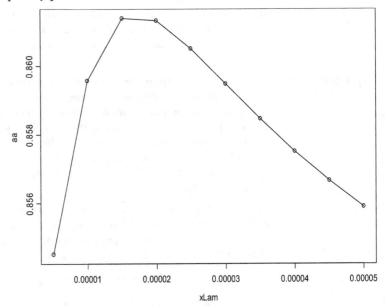

Figure 9.3: *Cross-validated correlations for six values of the penalty parameter.*

The third value of lambda (0.000015) maximizes the correlation, although that the correlations do not vary significantly over the values of lambda considered. We fit the final canonical correlations with lambda equal to 0.000015:

```
> gaitCancor <- fCancor(fGait[, 1], fGait[, 2],
                        xPenalty=list(lambda=0.000015,
```

```
                                        linDop=fDop(2)))
> par(mfrow=c(2, 1))
> plot(gaitCancor, main="Smoothed Result")
```

The result is displayed in Figure 9.4.

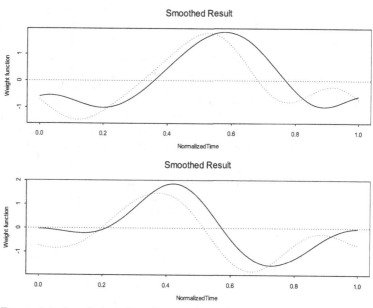

Figure 9.4: *Smoothed weighting functions for the first two canonical correlations. The solid curve corresponds to the hip data.*

The regularization gives a better (less optimistic) estimate of the first canonical correlation.

While cross validation is an effective means of estimating a penalty for the first canonical correlation, this penalty may not be appropriate for the remaining canonical correlations. Moreover, different penalties cannot be used for different levels of canonical correlation because of loss of orthogonality, so that in general determining more than one functional canonical correlations is not straightforward.

Interpreting the Coefficients

As in a functional principal component analysis, interpretation of the canonical correlation coefficient (weight) functions is important in understanding the analysis. The weight functions are normalized to

151

have *l*-2 norm (integral of the squared function) equal to 1. At each time point the weight function value is the weight that is given to the deviation of the function from the function mean.

From the top half of Figure 9.4, it is apparent that highly positive canonical scores for both the hip and knee curves tend to be less than the mean at both tails, and greater than the mean in the middle of the stride, while highly negative scores tend to be greater than the means in the tails, and less than the mean in the middle of the curve. The knee curve places more weight on the lower tail, with less weights on the upper tail. This may reflect a "locking" of the knee towards the end of the stride. This is illustrated by comparing the mean difference curves for the "middle" range of the positive values versus the "middle" negative values. The following code plots these differences on both the first, and the second, canonical variates:

```
> par(mfrow=c(2, 2))
> ii <- order(gaitCancor$variates[, 1, 1])
> plot(fVector(mean(fGait[, 1]), mean(fGait[ii[6:15], 1]),
        mean(fGait[ii[25:34], 1])), main="Can. 1, Hip")
> ii <- order(gaitCancor$variates[,1,2])
> plot(fVector(mean(fGait[, 2]), mean(fGait[ii[6:15], 2]),
        mean(fGait[ii[25:34], 2])), main="Can. 1, Knee")
> ii <- order(gaitCancor$variates[, 2, 1])
> plot(fVector(mean(fGait[, 1]), mean(fGait[ii[6:15], 1]),
        mean(fGait[ii[25:34], 1])), main="Can. 2, Hip")
> ii <- order(gaitCancor$variates[, 2, 2])
> plot(fVector(mean(fGait[, 2]), mean(fGait[ii[6:15], 2]),
        mean(fGait[ii[25:34], 2])), main="Can. 2, Knee")
```

The resulting plot is displayed in Figure 9.5.

In the hip curves for the first canonical correlation (upper left), the positive values for the canonical variate tend to be below the curve at the beginning and end of the cycle, and above the curve about halfway through the cycle, where the minimum hip angle is reached. These individuals show less of a swing in their hip movement than the average. The negative values for the canonical deviate show much the reverse, being above the curve at the beginning and end of the cycle, and reaching a smaller minimum than the average. The range of their hip angles tends to be larger than the average. Similar statements apply to the knee angle in canonical variate 1 (upper left): the positive canonical variates tend to have less extreme knee movement, while the negative values tend to have more extreme knee movement.

We now consider the second canonical variate in the second row of Figure 9.5. These curves are much like the two curves for the first canonical variate, except that there is much less variability in the early part of the curve - the variability is concentrated around 0.85 for the hip, where the positive canonical values show a smaller maximum than the negative canonical variate, and around 0.7 for the knee. Again, the positive variates show less of an extreme at this maximum than do the negative variates.

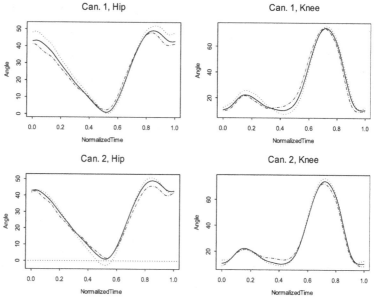

Figure 9.5: *The mean curve (solid line) mean curve for some positive (dashed line) and negative (dotted line) values of the canonical deviates.*

FUNCTIONAL CLUSTER ANALYSIS

10

Cluster analysis is an exploratory method used to find groups or clusters of similar data points. Classical *hierarchical* cluster analysis requires a matrix containing the distances between the items to be clustered. To compute a distance matrix, a *metric* or distance measure between any two data points is required. Functional methods offer many methods for computing distance matrixes, as was seen in Chapter 1, where the distance measure was taken as the integrated squared distance or l_2 distance between the two functions first derivatives.

Here we consider two examples involving daily measurements of precipitation and mean daily temperature at 35 Canadian weather stations over a one-year period. The functions provide an estimate of the expected daily temperatures at these stations. Ideally, additional years of observations would be desirable for analysis. We proceed by regularizing or smoothing the data, and then using the resulting functions to cluster the weather stations. As in the example in Chapter 1, the distance measure is obtained from the first derivatives of the smoothed functions.

CLUSTERING PRECIPITATION DATA

We first consider the daily precipitation data, and begin by smoothing the data using the construct function fVector. Daily precipitation is often highly variable with no precipitation on some days and a large amount of precipitation on others. Moreover, dry spells can last for quite some time, as can rainy periods. We are interested in the "expected" precipitation function, but we have only one year of measurements. Because we are interested in the first derivative function (the rate of change of the expected precipitation) and not in the measurement errors about the function, cross validation for these errors is not really helpful and we simply smooth until we seem to have an appropriate amount of smoothing by examining the first derivative of the smoothed function:

```
> sPrec <- fVector(fWeather$fPrec,
            penalty=list(lambda=100000, linDop=fDop(2)))
> par(mfrow=c(2, 1))
> plot(sPrec, main="Precipitation Functions")
> plot(fVector(sPrec, linDop=fDop(1)),
      main="Precipitation Derivatives")
```

In this code the unsmoothed precipitation functions are contained in the fPrec variable in the fWeather data frame (see the help file for fWeather). The smoothed functions are displayed in Figure 10.1. Looking at this Figure, the precipitation functions and their derivatives are reasonably smooth, giving a fairly good idea of the trend in the precipitation over the year that the data was measured.

Standardizing   Some patterns are evident in the expected precipitation functions, but precipitation is highly variable, depending to a considerable extent on local situations. For example, the western sides of mountains on the west coast of North America tend to get more rain as the weather station elevation increases (because of lifting), but the "trend" in weather variation is identical at all elevations. Because of this increase, we should be less interested in clustering based solely on the amount of precipitation, but rather on the rate of precipitation over the course of the year. Therefore, we standardize all weather stations to a fixed amount of fifty inches. This is accomplished by first integrating the smoothed precipitation functions over the year to get the total amount of precipitation, and then adjusting each function so that its integral is 50:

```
> precInt <- fInt(sPrec)/50
> ssPrec <- fVector(t(t(getCoef(sPrec))/precInt),
                    getBasis(sPrec), getNames(sPrec))
> par(mfrow=c(2, 1))
> plot(ssPrec, main="Standardized Precipitation")
> plot(fVector(ssPrec, linDop=fDop(1)), main=
        "Derivative of the Standardized Precipitation")
```

This result is displayed in Figure 10.2, which shows that the patterns of precipitation are now much more apparent. Indeed, some stations report the bulk of their precipitation over the winter months, while in others, most precipitation occurs in the summer.

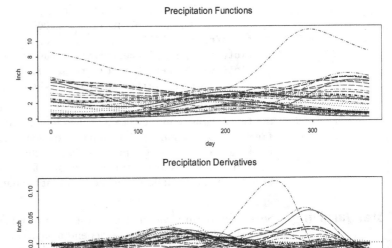

Figure 10.1: *Plot of the "expected" precipitation functions for 35 Canadian weather stations (top), with the first derivative (bottom).*

Clustering

To perform a hierarchical cluster analysis, we must first compute the between-station distance matrix using S+FDA function fDist. Here we use the integrated squared differences in the rate of change of precipitation as our clustering criterion. The S-PLUS function hclust is then used to cluster the data using a complete-linkage algorithm:

```
> ssPrecDist <- sqrt(fDist(ssPrec, linDop=fDop(1)))
> ssPrecClust <- hclust(ssPrecDist)
```

Standardized Precipitation

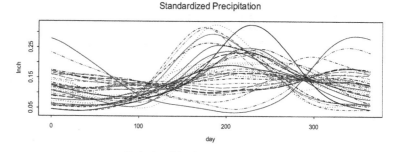

Derivative of the Standardized Precipitation

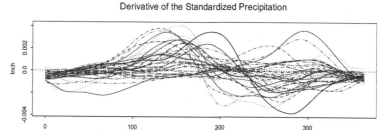

Figure 10.2: *The precipitation functions standardized to 50 inches per year.*

Complete linkage is chosen because we want the maximum within cluster distance to be small. Rather than plot the cluster tree, we plot the means of the seven cluster solution. The cutree function is used to identify stations within the seven clusters, as follows:

```
> ii <- cutree(ssPrecClust, k=7)
> ssPrecMean <- ssPrec[1:7]
> for(i in 1:7)
       ssPrecMean[i] <- mean(ssPrec[ii==i])
> par(mfrow=c(1, 1))
> plot(ssPrecMean,
```

```
                    main="Mean Functions for Seven Clusters")
     > legend(0, 0.325, as.character(1:7), lty=1:7)
```

The result is displayed in Figure 10.3, which shows that the cluster mean functions exhibit distinct patterns of precipitation.

Mean Functions for Seven Clusters

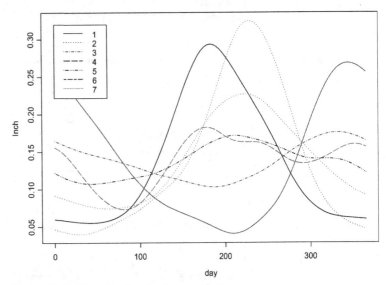

Figure 10.3: *Mean functions for the seven clusters.*

To see if the clustering result makes sense, we find the cities corresponding to the weather stations for each cluster:

- 1) Calgary, Edmonton, Prince Albert, Regina, The Pass, Winnipeg

- 2) Churchill, Dawson, Inuvik, Iqaluit, Schefferville, Thunder Bay, Uranium City, Whitehorse, Yellowknife

- 3) Charlottetown, Fredericton, Halifax, Prince Rupert, St. Johns, Sydney, Yarmouth

- 4) Kamloops, Prince George

- 5) Arvida, Bagotville, London, Montreal, Ottawa, Quebec, Sherbrooke, Toronto

- 6) Vancouver, Victoria

- 7) Resolute

Some of these results are expected, e.g., we would expect the far northern cities in cluster 2 to be similar, and Vancouver and Victoria, both in cluster 6, clearly share the same weather pattern being less that fifty miles apart and separated only by a body of water. On the other hand, we have no reason to believe that Halifax, on the east coast, and Prince Rupert, on the west coast, would have the same weather patterns, although they are both coastal cities. Clearly clustering based upon precipitation patterns is useful in finding groups of weather stations with related weather patterns, but precipitation patterns alone are insufficient to characterize the weather data.

CLUSTERING TEMPERATURE DATA

We now consider the temperature data. Unlike the precipitation data, here we do not standardize to a constant mean temperature. We look at the rate of change of the average daily temperature, rather than at the expected average daily temperature function. As with the precipitation data, smoothing is used to obtain an "expected" daily temperature from a single year of data.

The S+FDA statements used to smooth the data, perform a cluster analysis, and compute and plot the cluster mean functions are as follows:

```
> sTemp <- fVector(fWeather$fTemp,
                penalty=list(lambda=50000, linDop=fDop(2)))
> sTempDist <- sqrt(fDist(sTemp, linDop=fDop(1)))
> sTempClust <- hclust(sTempDist)
> jj <- cutree(sTempClust, k=7)
> sTempMean <- sTemp[1:7]
> for(i in 1:7)
        sTempMean[i] <- mean(sTemp[jj==i])
> par(mfrow=c(2,1))
> plot(sTempMean, main=
        "Temperature Cluster Mean Functions")
> plot(fVector(sTempMean), main=
        "Derivatives of Temperature Cluster Mean Functions")
> legend(300, 0.4, as.character(1:7), lty=1:7)
```

The result is shown in Figure 10.4.

The temperature-based clusters are composed of the following stations. Here the number in parenthesis is the cluster number for the plot legend.

1. (3) Calgary, Edmonton, Kamloops, Prince George, Whitehorse

2. (1) Dawson, Prince Albert, Regina, The Pas, Uranium City, Winnipeg, Yellowknife

3. (6) Charlottetown, Halifax, St. Johns, Sydney, Yarmouth

4. (5) Churchill, Iqaluit, Schefferville

5. (4) Arvida, Bagotville, Fredericton, London, Montreal, Ottawa,

Quebec, Sherbrooke, Thunder Bay, Toronto

6. (7) Prince Rupert, Vancouver, Victoria

7. (2) Inuvik, Resolute

Again there are stations whose cluster assignment make sense (e.g., cluster 6 (7)), as well as clusters which are difficult to interpret (e.g, cluster 2 (1)).

Temperature Cluster Mean Functions

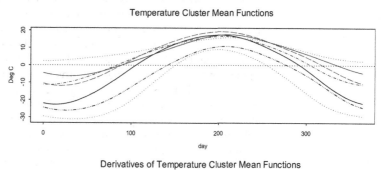

Derivatives of Temperature Cluster Mean Functions

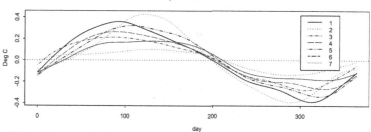

Figure 10.4: *The cluster mean functions for temperature (top) and its derivative (bottom).*

SUMMARY

Cluster analysis is an exploratory technique. Functional data methods offer the advantage of allowing a greater variety of clustering matrixes to choose from. The examples involving the clustering of Canadian weather stations are meant to be illustrative, since the known locations of weather stations can be used to infer which ones should exhibit similar weather patterns. The objective is not so much to find "real" clusters of stations, but rather to learn how the weather patterns at the different stations are related. Some of the clusters obtained consist of stations that are located in the same region, which we would expect similar to have weather patterns. Other aspects of the clustering are harder to interpret (e.g., assignment of Prince Rupert and Halifax to the same cluster), although they may also indicate relationships in weather patterns for stations at some distance from each other. A cluster analysis that accounted for both precipitation and temperature (and other weather related variables such as humidity) might be preferable, provided a suitable clustering metric could be found.

Methods for determining the number of clusters in functional cluster analysis are identical to those in the classical case, and thus are not discussed further here.

If groupings for some of the data are known in advance, it may be preferable to use a discriminant function analysis to find the variables and matrix that best classify the remaining observations. In the chapter on functional generalized linear models, we use a form of discriminant function analysis, functional logistic models, to classify the weather stations.

PRINCIPAL DIFFERENTIAL
ANALYSIS

11

Principal differential analysis (Ramsay 1996) estimates linear systems of ordinary differential equations approximately satisfied by functional data. This is of interest in physical processes, where, for example, the one-dimensional motion of an object is a function of time that solves an ordinary differential equation. The Maxwell equations are another well known physical example. Biological, chemical and other phenomena also often satisfy ordinary differential equations, and discovering the form of these equations can help to understand the nature of the underlying process.

More formally, for a sample of functions $f_j(t), j = 1, ..., n$, principal differential analysis determines a linear differential operator L of degree m and/or a function $\alpha(t)$ for which $Lf_j(t) \approx \alpha(t)$ for all j. Here L is defined as:

$$L = \sum_{i=0}^{m} \beta_i(t)D^i$$

where the operator notation has the following interpretation:

$$D^0 f_j(t) = f_j(t) \text{ and } D^i f_j(t) = \frac{d^i f_j(t)}{dt^i}, \text{ the } i^{\text{th}} \text{ derivative of } f_j(t).$$

In principal, both the forcing function $\alpha(t)$ and the linear differential operator weights (coefficients) $\beta_i(t)$ may be functional data objects. However, the current implementation may not be reliable unless the linear differential operator is known to have constant coefficients. Methods that better handle more general linear differential operators are under active research, and will be added to S+FDA in the future.

Given the form of $\alpha(t)$ and the $\beta_i(t)$, the linear differential equation is estimated by least squares (or penalized least squares). Either $\alpha(t)$ or one of the $\beta_i(t)$ must be known. Computational procedures are discussed in Chapter 14 of Ramsay and Silverman (1997). Penalized least squares estimation minimizes the criterion:

which reduces to a least squares criterion if the penalty term is omitted.

$$\sum_{j=1}^{n} \int [Lf_j(s) - \alpha(s)]^2 ds + penalty$$

The function $\alpha(t)$ is called the *forcing* function since, when $m = 2$, it corresponds to the external force applied to a physical system. If $\alpha(t)$ is identically zero, the resulting differential equation is said to be *homogeneous*. Otherwise the system is *nonhomogeneous*.

When the forcing function $\alpha(t)$ and/or weight functions $\beta_i(t)$ are unknown, principal differential analysis can be used to estimate them and elucidate the process underlying the functions $f_j(t)$.

Like principal components, principal differential analysis allows re-expressing the functional data in terms of a set of basis functions that may be considerably more compact than the current representation. This follows from the fact that all solutions to a linear differential equation can be expressed as the sum of:

- a particular solution

and

- a linear combination of basis functions for the null space or *kernel* of the linear differential operator.

Although the current implementation of S+FDA cannot currently handle arbitrary bases, such a representation may nevertheless be useful in an analysis.

S+FDA FUNCTIONS FOR PRINCIPAL DIFFERENTIAL ANALYSIS

The S+FDA function fPDA estimates the weight functions $\beta_i(t)$ for the linear differential operator L, and/or the forcing function, $\alpha(t)$. The fPDA object is a list with two components:

- an object of class fLinDop which gives the coefficients of the estimated linear differential operator.

- an object of class fFunction which gives the estimated forcing function.

The fPDA object also has fitted.values and residuals from predictions of the original functional data as attributes.

There is a predict method for fPDA objects that calls a function fLinDopSolve to solve the linear differential equation. The fitting for prediction is done by linear regression involving the kernel basis functions of the linear differential operator and a particular solution to the differential equation if there is a nonzero forcing function. See Ramsay and Silverman (1997) for more details.

RADIOACTIVE DECAY EXAMPLE

Consider radioactive decay defined by

$$y'(t) = -ky(t)$$

where $y(t)$ is the amount of a chemical element present at time t, k is the rate constant intrinsic to the element, and $y'(t)$ is the rate of decay. The linear differential operator is:

$$L = D^{(1)} + kD^{(0)}$$

The goal is to estimate k.

To illustrate the S+FDA principal differential analysis function, fPDA, we construct an example of functional data described by the above radioactive decay equation. We simulate data for iodine 131, for which $k = 0.0864$ when the unit of time is days.

```
> rateConstantI131 <- 0.0864
> Time <- 0:50
> Y <- matrix(0, 51, 10)
> set.seed(0) # seed for reproducing random numbers
> for(j in 1:10)
      Y[,j] <- (100 + rnorm(1, sd=10))*
                      exp(rateConstantI131*Time)
```

Since the differential equation is of order one, we use a B-spline basis of order four so that the first derivative will be a smooth cubic spline.

```
> basis <- bsplineBasis(c(0,50), norder=4, nbasis=10)
```

The functional data object created from the basis is:

```
> fY <- fVector(basis, Y)
```

Plot the functional data (see Figure 11.1:):

```
> par(mfrow=c(1, 1))
> plot(fY, main="Radioactive Decay of Iodine 131")
```

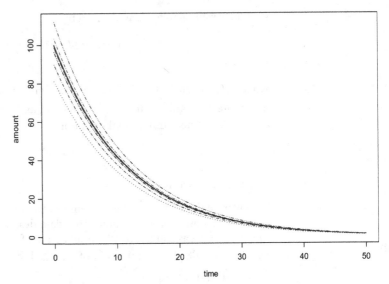

Figure 11.1: *Functional data for radioactive decay of Iodine 131.*

To estimate the rate constant, we first call fPDA.

```
> decayPDAconst <-
        fPDA(fY, weights=list(constantBasis(fDomain=
                               c(0, 50)), 1), forcing=0)
```

Here we have set weights=list(constantBasis(fDomain= c(0,50)), 1) to indicate that the first order coefficient is known to be equal to 1, and the zeroth order coefficient needs to be estimated. We use a constantBasis to ensure that the estimated coefficient is a constant.

The value of the rate constant estimate is then given as follows:

```
> rateConstantEstimate <-
                  fEval(decayPDAconst$linDop[[1]], 25)
> rateConstantEstimate
            [,1]
[1,] 0.08638197
```

(since the coefficient is constant it suffices to evaluate the weight function at any point in the domain).

The following code plots the original functional data object, the predictions produced by `predict.fPDA`, the residuals from the predictions, and the operator residuals (Lf):

```
> predictions <- predict(decayPDAconst)
> par(mfrow=c(2, 2))
> plot(fY, main="Original Functional Data")
> plot(predictions$fitted,
        main="Predicted Functional Data")
> plot(predictions$residuals,
        main="Residuals of Predicted Values")
> Lx <- fEval(fY, fArg=Time, linDop=decayPDAconst$linDop)
> plot(fVector(getBasis(fY), y=Lx),
        main="Differential Operator Residuals")
```

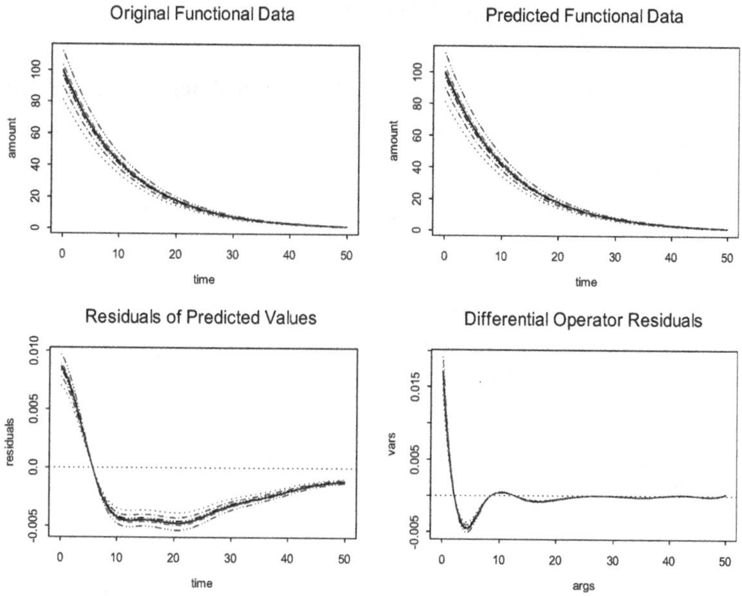

Figure 11.2: *Functional data, predicted fitted values, residuals of predicted values, and operator residuals, when constant coefficients are assumed.*

In the example just given, we chose a constant basis because of the theoretical equation of decay. But it may be of interest to know what fPDA would estimate if we did not make this assumption.

```
> decayPDAvar <- fPDA(fY, weights=list(NULL, 1), forcing=0)
```

171

Setting the first element of weights to `NULL` causes the basis of the functional data `fY` to be used in estimating the forcing function. More generally, a basis can be specified for each unknown function in the linear differential equation.

Plot the estimated rate of decay.

```
> plot(decayPDAvar$linDop[[1]],
        ylab="Decay Rate Estimate", xlab="Domain",
        main="Decay Rate Estimate, using inherited basis")
> abline(h=-0.0864)
```

Figure 11.3: shows that on average the estimated rate of decay is close to the theoretical rate. However, there are edge effects, hinting at the difficulties to be encountered in situations where less is known about the underlying process, and one or more coefficients are estimated using a nonconstant basis.

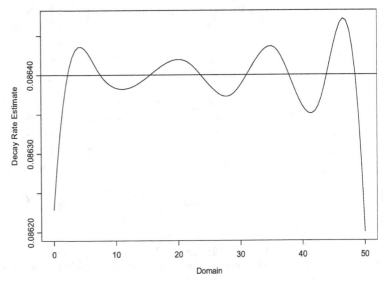

Decay Rate Estimate, using inherited basis

Figure 11.3: *Estimated rate of decay, using the basis of the functional data object. The horizontal line is drawn at the theoretical decay rate.*

HARMONIC OSCILLATOR EXAMPLE

A mechanical system is characterized by an external force applied to the system, together with internal or external frictional forces or viscosity. The classic example is a weight suspended from a spring. The spring will oscillate when the weight is attached to it provided the weight is not too heavy. This motion will fade over time depending on the viscosity of the air or other medium in which the system is situated.

The equation of motion for a harmonic oscillator with external force f is:

$$D^2 y + k_1 Dy + k_0 y = f$$

where k_1 is the damping constant and k_0 is the square of the natural oscillating frequency.

Underdamped + Resonance

The second-order equation of motion describes an *underdamped* system if $k_1 < 2\sqrt{k_0}$. In this case, oscillation will occur. If the forcing function exhibits periodicty, the oscillation is called *resonance*. An analytic solution is known when the forcing function is of the form $C\cos(2\pi v t)$, where $2\pi v$ is the resonance frequency. A particular solution in this case is

$$A\sin(2\pi v t) + B\cos(2\pi v t)$$

A general solution to the differential equation can be obtained by adding the particular solution to the homogeneous solution, which (ignoring the phase shift) is

$$C\exp\left(-k_1 \frac{t}{2}\right)\sin(t\sqrt{k_0})$$

under the assumption that the system is underdamped. The following code simulates such a system and plots the resulting functional data:

```
> k0 <- 2
> k1 <- .5
> hconst <- fconst <- 10
> phase <- 0
> nu <- 1/3

> pi2nu <- 2*pi*nu
> a <- pi2nu*k1
> b <- k0 - pi2nu*pi2nu
> d <- a*a + b*b
> A <- a/d
> B <- b/d

> tt <- seq(from=0, to=5, length=101)
> Y <- matrix(0, 101, 10)
> set.seed(0) # seed for reproducing random numbers
> for(j in 1:10)
    Y[,j] <- hconst*exp(-k1*tt/2)*sin(sqrt(k0)*tt+phase) +
        fconst*(A*sin(pi2nu*tt) + B*cos(pi2nu*tt)) + rnorm(1)
```

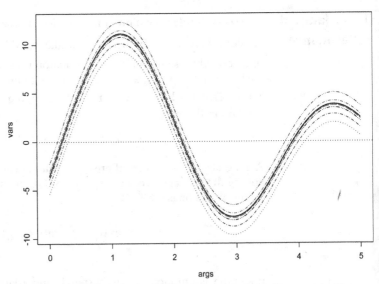

Figure 11.4: *Simulated functional data for an underdamped harmonic oscillator with resonance.*

Now we compute the constant coefficients of the linear differential
operator assuming that the forcing function is known:

```
> par(mfrow=c(1, 1))
> basis <- bsplineBasis(c(0, 5), norder=5, nbasis=20)
> fY <- fVector(basis, Y)
> plot(fY, main="Underdamped + Resonance")

# compute constant coeffs using known forcing function
> forcing <- fFunction(basis, fconst * cos(pi2nu*tt))
> oscPDAconst <- fPDA(fY, weights=
                        list(constantBasis(c(0, 5)),
                             constantBasis(c(0, 5)), 1),
                        forcing=forcing)
> k0 <- fEval(oscPDAconst$linDop[[1]], 2.5)
> k0
          [,1]
[1,] 2.021411
> k1 <- fEval(oscPDAconst$linDop[[2]], 2.5)
> k1
           [,1]
[1,] 0.504323
```

The resulting coefficients are quite close to the true values underlying
the simulated data.

In this case fPDA also gives a good estimate of the forcing function
when the linear differential operator is known:

```
> oscPDAforc <- fPDA(fY, weights=list(2, .5, 1),
                        forcing=basis)
> plot(ans1$forcing, main="Estimated Forcing Function
                           (known LDO)")
> lines(tt, fEval(forcing, tt), lty=6)
```

Estimated Forcing Function (known LDO)

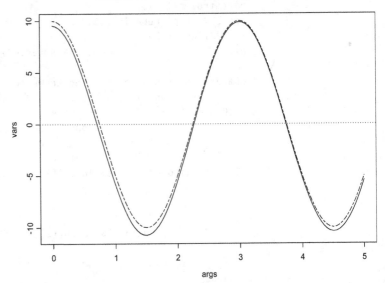

Figure 11.5: *Forcing function for underdamped harmonic oscillator estimated by fPDA when the linear differential operator is known. The dotted line is the true forcing function underlying the simulated data.*

However, if we attempt to estimate the linear differential operator coefficients as well as the forcing function, the resulting least squares problem is ill-conditioned.

```
> oscPDAall <- fPDA(fY, weights=list(constantBasis(c(0,5)),
                    constantBasis(c(0, 5)), 1),forcing=basis)
Warning in fPDA(fY, weights = list(constantBasis(c(..:
                    least-squares system is ill-conditioned
```

The ill-conditioning warning is usually means that the results will not be accurate, as is the case for this example. The constant weights are estimated to be 0 and 0.083, far from their true values of 2 and 0.5, respectively. The forcing function estimate is plotted below:

```
> plot(oscPDAall$forcing, main="Forcing Function Estimate")
```

```
> lines(tt, fEval(forcing, tt), lty=6)
```

Forcing Function Estimate

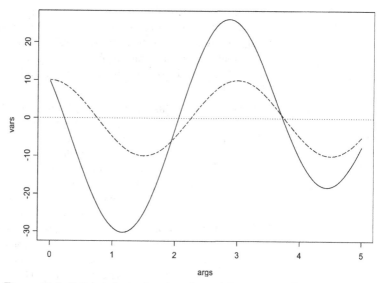

Figure 11.6: *Estimate forcing function when weights are assumed constant but unknown. The dotted line is the true forcing function underlying the simulated data.*

It may in some instances be possible to avoid ill-conditioning by increasing the arguments k or nbasis to fPDA (these affect the accuracy of the projections used in computing inner products for least squares), but in this case we weren't able to find a suitable set of inputs. It is also possible to include penalty terms on the weight functions and/or their derivatives, or on the derivatives of the forcing function, in fPDA to regularize principal differential analysis, but there are no systematic guidelines for doing so with the current implementation. New methods under development incorporate regularization mechanisms, and we plan to include them in future editions of this library.

LIP MOVEMENT EXAMPLE

The lip movement data, first used in the chapter on registration, consists of twenty replications measuring the vertical lip position as a single individual says the syllable "bob". In order to perform principal differential analysis, first register and smooth the curves. The S+FDA code for creating, registering, and smoothing the lip data is as follows:

```
> lipBasis <- fBasis(type="bspline",fDomain=c(0, 1),
                     nbasis=31,params=(c(1:25)/26))
> fLip <- fVector(object=lipBasis, y=lipmat, fArgs=liptime,
                  fNames=list(NormalizedTime=liptime,
                  Replications=seq(20), Units="mm"))
> regLip1 <- fRegister(fLip, mean(fLip), nDeriv=1,
                       maxIter=120, lambda=0.1,
                       criterion=1, penalty=0.0005)
> regLip1 <- fRegister(fLip,mean(regLip1$fReg), nDeriv=1,
                       maxIter=120, lambda=0.1,
                       criterion=1, penalty=0.0005)
> yLip <- fVector(regLip1$fReg, penalty=
                  list(lambda=1.e-10, linDop=fDop(2)))
```

Note in this code that the registration is performed on the derivatives rather than the functions.

Because the lower lip is part of a mechanical system, with certain natural resonance frequencies and a stiffness or resistance to movement, it seems appropriate to explore to what extent this method can be expressed it terms of the second-order differential equation typically used to analyze such systems, in which the linear differential operator

$$\beta_0(t)f(t) + \beta_1(t)D^1f(t) + D^2f(t)$$

is a generalization of the which one used for the harmonic oscillator example in the previous section. Strictly speaking, the mechanical interpretation of the differential equations does not hold if the weight coefficients are allowed to be functions rather than constants, but higher-order effects can be ignored if they do not vary too rapidly with time. The principal differential analysis estimates, assuming nonconstant weights, are computed as follows:

```
> lipPDA <- fPDA(yLip, weights=list(NULL, NULL, 1),
                 forcing=0)
```

We set `forcing=0` to indicate that the differential equation is assumed to be homogeneous (no forcing function). A plot of the residuals for the homogeneous fit with the weight functions estimated by `fPDA`, as given in Figure 11.7:, is calculated as follows.

```
> lipPDA <- fPDA(yLip, weights=list(NULL, NULL, 1),
                 forcing=0)
# calculate and plot residual Lx
> lipResiduals <- fEval(yLip, fArg=liptime,
                        linDop=lipPDA$linDop)

> keep <- liptime >= 0.1 & liptime <= 0.9
> matplot(liptime[keep], lipResiduals[keep,], type="l")
```

Points at the ends of the plot have been removed in order to eliminate edge effects near 0 and 1.

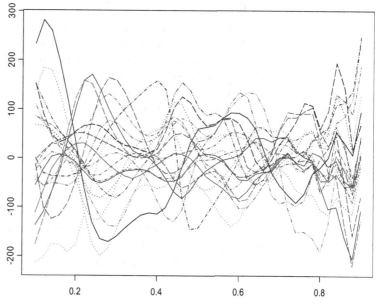

Figure 11.7: *Operator residuals from the second-order differential equation fit to the lip movement data.*

Although the residual results are not nearly as small as we would prefer (for comparison, the largest magnitude of the second derivatives is near 500), they still appear to be more or less random, indicating that the linear differential operator is capturing the functional behavior.

Kernel Basis Functions

Like principal components, principal differential analysis allows re-expressing the functional data in terms of a set of coefficients that may be much smaller than the current representation. Although the current implementation of S+FDA does not allow arbitrary bases, this property may still be useful in an analysis.

Specifically, if L is a linear differential operator of degree m, then there are m linearly independent functions $u_1, u_2, ..., u_m$ (the *kernel basis functions*) that span the null space or *kernel* of L, that is, for which $Lu_i = 0$. The kernel basis functions are determined by m constraints, which may include initial conditions and/or boundary conditions.

In the theory of linear ordinary differential equations, all solutions to the homogeneous equation are linear combinations of the kernel basis functions. If the weight functions defining L are determined by principal differential analysis, and residuals for the ordinary differential equation are small, then for homogeneous equations there should be a linear combination of the form

$$f_j(t) = \sum_{i=1}^{m} \gamma_{ij} u_i(t) + \varepsilon_j(t)$$

in which the residual terms $\varepsilon_j(t)$ are relatively small.

For nonhomogeneous equations, any solution can be expressed as the sum of a particular solution and a linear combination of the kernel basis functions. So if $x(t)$ is a particular solution, then the functional data have the following representation:

$$f_j(t) = x(t) + \sum_{i=1}^{m} \gamma_{ij} u_i(t) + \varepsilon_j(t)$$

Since each of the observed functions $f_j(t)$ is a solution, up to a random error, then the average function, $\overline{f(t)} = \frac{1}{n} \sum_{j=1}^{n} f_j(t)$ is also a solution with a random error, but the random error for $\overline{f(t)}$ is n times smaller than for each function $f_j(t)$. Thus, when the errors are small, $\overline{f(t)}$ approximates a particular solution to the differential equation, and consequently a good fit of the centered functions $f_j(t) - \overline{f(t)}$ can be obtained as a linear combination of the kernel basis functions. Notice the similarity with functional principal components analysis, which finds a set of (orthogonal) functions that can be used to re-express the functions $f_j(t)$ such that the integrated squared error $\varepsilon_j(t)$ is minimized.

Change of Basis

A set of kernel basis functions, $u_1, u_2, ..., u_m$ for a linear differential operator can be computed via the function fLinDopSolve:

```
> lipKernData <- fLinDopSolve(linDop=lipPDA$linDop,
                              x=liptime)
> lipKern <- fVector(lipKernData, basis=getBasis(yLip))
> par(mfrow=c(2, 1))
> plot(lipKern[1], main="First Kernel Basis Function")
> plot(lipKern[2], main="Second Kernel Basis Function")
```

The resulting basis is displayed in Figure 11.8. Notice that the first kernel basis function has a much larger range than the second one indicating, perhaps, that the first basis function is more important.

First Kernel Basis Function

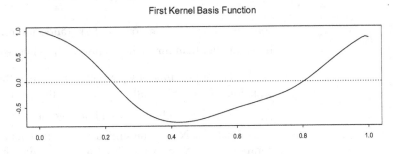

Second Kernel Basis Function

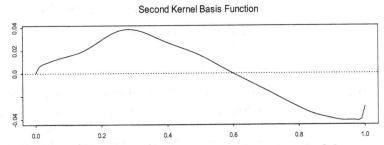

Figure 11.8: *Kernel basis functions for the linear differential operator fit by principal differential analysis to the lip force data.*

The S+FDA function fLinDopSolve is based on the adaptive ordinary differential equation solvers DLSODA and DLSODI (Hindmarsh 1983; Petzold 1983). Initial conditions may be specified through the initialValues argument. Different initial conditions can lead to different kernel basis functions, but all sets of kernel basis functions span the same function space and are thus equivalent for our purposes.

Given the kernel basis functions for a linear differential operator, the function fLinDopFit can be used to obtain a representation of a function in terms of the kernel basis. Below we compute this fit for the lip motion data, from which the linear differential operator was derived.

```
> lipFit <- fLinDopFit(yLip, linDop=lipPDA$linDop)
> par(mfrow=c(2, 1))
```

```
> plot(lipFit$fitted.values, main="Fitted Values")
> plot(lipFit$residuals, main="Residual Functions")
```

The fit is accomplished via least-squares projection of the observed functions onto the kernel basis. The fitted functions and the residuals for the registered lip movement functions are displayed in Figure 11.9. Note the difference between these residuals and those shown in Figure 11.7, which displays values of the linear differential operator applied to yLip, which are viewed as "residuals" when homogeneity is assumed.

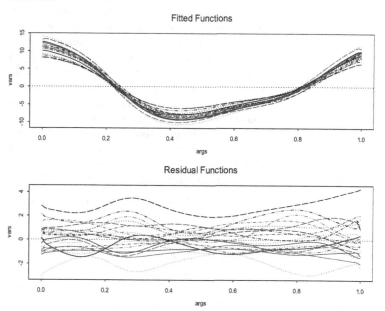

Figure 11.9: *Lip curves and residuals from the fit of the lip motion data to the kernel basis functions for the linear differential operator determined by fPDA.*

The fitted curves appear to be quite similar to the registered and smoothed lip curve functions, although the residual functions indicate that the fit is not perfect. Nevertheless, these residual functions are relatively small, with a range of about 25% of the range of the lip curves proper.

The residuals and fitted values given above are precisely those that would be obtained from predict applied to lipPDA, because the linear differential operator and data input to fLinDopFit came from

183

the principal differential analysis. Function fLinDopFit differs from the predict method for fPDA objects in that instead of an fPDA object it takes as input a linear differential operator and (optionally) a forcing function, and returns the predictors (kernel basis functions) and coefficients from the fit as well as the fitted values and residuals.

Comparison with PCA

Because of its relationship to functional principal components, it is useful to compare the fit obtained from the kernel basis functions obtained with the homogeneous functions with the fit obtained using a functional principal components analysis. Here we use the integrated residual variance as a measure of "goodness of fit". This statistic has meaning for both the functional principal components solution and for the functional principal differential analysis solutions, but is minimized in the functional principal components models - we expect, apriori, that principal differential analysis will not do as well as the principal component analysis in predicting variation in our lip movement data (if the same number of "parameters" are estimated). However, if the principal differential analysis solution explains a good deal of the functions variance, then we would have some evidence that the estimated linear differential equation has the correct form and closely models the process that generated the data.

In the following code we compute the harmonics using function fPCA as well as the fitted values for fPDA, and computed the integrated variance using functions fInt and fVar.

```
> ansPCA <- fPCA(~yLip)
> phi <- double(3)
> phi[1] <- fInt(fVar(yLip, bivariate=F))
> phi[2] <- fInt(fVar(fVector(getCoef(yLip)
            -outer(c(getCoef(mean(yLip))), rep(1, 20))
            -getCoef(ansPCA$harmonics) %*% t(ansPCA$scores),
            getBasis(yLip)), bivariate=F))
> phi[3] <- fInt(fVar(predict(lipPDA)$residuals,
                      bivariate=F))

> par(mfrow=c(1, 1))
> plot(fVar(yLip, bivariate=F), xlab="t", ylab="Var(f(t))",
        main="Variance Functions", ylim=c(0,5))
> lines(fVar(fVector(getCoef(yLip)
          - outer(c(getCoef(mean(yLip))), rep(1,20))
          - getCoef(ansPCA$harmonics) %*% t(ansPCA$scores),
```

```
        getBasis(yLip)),bivariate=F), lty=2)
> lines(fVar(predict(lipPDA)$residuals, bivariate=F),
        lty=3)
> legend(0.6, 5, c("Mean", "PCA", "PDA"), lty=1:3)
```

The plot of the variance functions shown in Figure 11.10:.

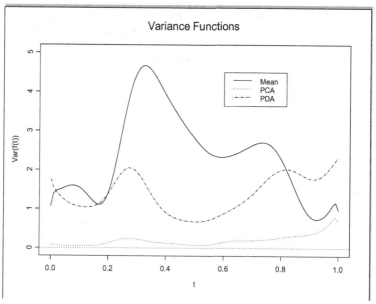

Figure 11.10: *Variance functions for PCA and PDA analyses of the lip motion data.*

Finally, we compute an "r-squared"-like measure for goodness of fit based upon these integrated variances:

```
> Rsq <- 1-phi[2:3]/phi[1]
> names(Rsq) <- c("PCA", "PDA")
> Rsq
     PCA        PDA
 0.9147264 0.4107527
```

From both the R-squared statistics and the variance function plots we see that the two harmonic functional principal component solution provides the best fit, as expected.

Summary

An unique aspect of functional data analysis is its ability to provide insight into the processes underlying the functional data. The goal of principal differential analysis - to find an underlying differential equation describing the behavior a sample of observations - is an exciting and powerful idea. The simple least-squares approach currently implemented in S+FDA is limited in what it can handle. However, new iterative approaches under development for principal differential analysis show great promise for improvement, and in the next release of this library, we expect to significantly enhance the methods provided here.

APPENDIX: REFERENCES

de Boor, C. (1978). *A Practical Guide to Splines*, Springer, New York.

Friedman, J. H. and B. W. Silverman (1989). Flexible parsimonious smoothing and additive modeling (Discussion and Response), *Journal of the American Statistical Association*, **31**, 1-39.

Green, P. J., and B. W. Silverman (1994). *Nonparametric Regression and Generalized Linear Models: A Roughness Penalty Approach*, Chapman and Hall, London.

Gu, Chong (2002). *Smoothing Spline ANOVA Models, Springer Series in Statistics*, Springer, New Youk.

Hollig, Klaus (2003). *Finite Element Methods with B-Splines*, SIAM, Philadelphia.

Kahaner, David, Cleve Moler, and Stephen Nash (1989). *Numerical Methods and Software*, Prentice Hall, Englewood Cliffs, New Jersey.

Matflat Nicole and Ramsay, J. O. (2003). *The Historical Functional Linear Model, The Canidian Journal of Statistics,* Vol. 31, No. 2, 115-128.

Lachenbruch, P. A. (1975), *Discriminant Analysis*, Hafner Press, New York.

Olshen, R. A., E. N. Biden, M.P. Wyatt, and D. H. Sutherland (1989). Gait analysis and the bootstrap, *Annals of Statistics*, **17**, 1419-1440.

Ramsay, J. O. and B. Silverman (1997). *Functional Data Analysis*, Springer-Verlag, New York.

Ramsay, J. O. and B. Silverman (2002). *Applied Functional Data Analysis*, Springer-Verlag, New York.

INDEX

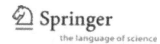
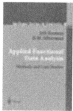
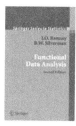